HEALTH CARE IN CRISIS

Health Care in Crisis

*Hospitals, Nurses, and the Consequences
of Policy Change*

Theresa Morris

NEW YORK UNIVERSITY PRESS

New York

NEW YORK UNIVERSITY PRESS
New York
www.nyupress.org

References to Internet websites (URLs) were accurate at the time of writing. Neither the author nor New York University Press is responsible for URLs that may have expired or changed since the manuscript was prepared.

Library of Congress Cataloging-in-Publication Data
Names: Morris, Theresa, 1956– author.
Title: Health care in crisis : hospitals, nurses, and the consequences of policy change / Theresa Morris.
Description: New York : New York University Press, [2018] | Includes bibliographical references and index.
Identifiers: LCCN 2017034390 | ISBN 978-1-4798-1352-0 (cl : alk. paper) | ISBN 978-1-4798-2769-5 (pb : alk. paper)
Subjects: LCSH: Medical economics—United States. | Medical care—United States.
Classification: LCC RA410.53 .M664 2018 | DDC 338.4/73621—dc23
LC record available at https://lccn.loc.gov/2017034390

New York University Press books are printed on acid-free paper, and their binding materials are chosen for strength and durability. We strive to use environmentally responsible suppliers and materials to the greatest extent possible in publishing our books.

Manufactured in the United States of America

10 9 8 7 6 5 4 3 2 1

Also available as an ebook

This book is dedicated to my mom, Susan, and the memory of my dad, Gary Michael, and of my Aunt Mary, the first nurse I ever knew.

CONTENTS

Introduction

How does a hospital—a complex organization that coordinates health-promoting and life-saving services provided by hundreds of workers amid ever-changing science and technology—respond to rapid and sweeping policy changes that upend how it all gets paid for? Below are excerpts from interviews I conducted with a nurse and an administrator that indicate two extreme views of the impact of such changes on the obstetric unit of Fuller Hospital,[1] a small, non-profit, community hospital in New England:

> I had to call [the nurse manager] in tears one night . . . It was one o'clock in the morning, and . . . I'm in a room getting an epidural [for a patient], and I had three more patients [coming] in . . . I called [the nurse manager], and I said, "I can't take care of what's coming." . . . And that's a really terrible thing to feel like there's nothing else you can do. (Jamie, Fuller Hospital obstetrical nurse)

> I think it's definitely a challenge to go forward with . . . so many unknowns. I very firmly believe that community hospitals have to have that affiliation with a larger entity in order to be able to survive in the Accountable Care kind of world. . . . I am grateful that our board and our senior administration were so forward thinking that they started approaching a partnership before we got to a place of financial desperation. (Joyce, administrator of Fuller Hospital obstetric unit)[2]

Both the administrator and nurse are dealing with changes Fuller Hospital is facing because of federal and state health-care policy changes. The national policy change that swept through the country in the 2013–16 period examined in this book is the Patient Protection and Affordable Care Act, more commonly referred to as the Affordable Care Act (ACA) or simply Obamacare. This book explores the experience of nurses in the obstetric (OB) unit of Fuller Hospital during this time of turbulent health-care policy change. The administrator in the excerpt above is looking forward to changes in the hospital as a strategy to deal with health-care policy changes; Jamie, an obstetrical (OB) nurse at Fuller Hospital, is living with the consequences of those changes—fewer support staff, more patients per nurse, and an endlessly busy unit. This book examines that tension.

* * *

Health-care provision in the United States has a history of being contentious.[3] As such, the ACA is part of a much-debated shift in U.S. policy that began in the 1970s in which the federal government began to intervene in health services in order to bring health-care costs under control.[4] The way that U.S. health-care policy has changed since has been influenced by this policy trajectory, the spread of large corporations in the health-care industry, and the ideology and behavior of what Paul Starr refers to as reprivatization in which public services are transferred to the ownership and/or control of private corporations.[5] In other words, the ACA cannot be separated from the historical roots of how the United States has dealt with health-care provision and payment. Thus, although the ACA stands out as a policy that instituted sweeping change, it stayed within the confines of privatized health care with only a public option, rather than a fully public system of health-care provision.[6] Further, because health-care provision is *so* contentious in the United States, the future of the ACA is unclear as of 2017, as I am writing. However, regardless of the ongoing health-care-provision saga, which, no doubt, will continue beyond the publication of this book, the arguments I present should be seen as an example of how rapid health-care policy change affects patients and nurses, rather than only a study of these *specific* policy changes' ramifications.

Let me begin with a very brief overview of how the ACA changed the health-care landscape. The most noted and talked about effect of the ACA is the spread of health insurance coverage to previously uninsured individuals. For example, according to the Congressional Budget Office and the Joint Committee on Taxation, between the enactment of the ACA in March 2010 and February 2016, the number of non-elderly Americans who have health insurance increased by twenty million, a change that, no doubt, benefits both society and those newly insured individuals.[7] A less talked about but still important goal of the ACA is to lower health-care costs through a change in clinician and hospital Medicare and Medicaid compensation.[8] For instance, since October 2012, hospitals have been assessed on quality measures such as readmissions and patient satisfaction, and federal reimbursements are now tied to hospitals' performance on these measures.[9] Further, on January 1, 2013, Medicare began incentive payments to hospitals that meet certain performance measures. This program was funded by *decreasing* existing Medicare payments by 1 percent, with the decrease in payments accelerating to 2 percent in 2017.[10] These changes in the structure of Medicare and Medicaid payments put new pressure on hospitals, especially small hospitals with few resources, to meet stepped-up standards of care. A common hospital response to this pressure is to partner with a larger and often for-profit health system or hospital that can contribute additional financial capital.

In this book I examine Fuller Hospital, a nearly one-hundred-year old, small, non-profit, community hospital in New England. After so many years of being a community health provider, Fuller Hospital sought an acquisition partner and was acquired by a for-profit hospital system, Waranoke Heath System, on October 1, 2016, after a failed acquisition attempt by a partnership between Axiom Health System, a for-profit health system, and Elite University in 2015. The hospital's board deliberately sought an acquisition to deal with financial pressures that administrators claimed came from policy changes, specifically the ACA and changes in state-level health-care policy. I studied OB nurses in Fuller Hospital from July 2013, when the administration was actively seeking an acquisition partner, through June 2016, just before a second acquisition attempt was set to close, to see how the period of rapid change affected the nurses and how they cared for patients.

I became interested in studying this topic because of my longstanding interest in the social determinants of women's reproductive health. I have studied how reality television programs inaccurately represent contemporary labor and birth by dramatizing and problematizing women's experiences.[11] I have also examined women's experiences with epidurals and cesareans and explored how these experiences differ by race.[12] However, what drew me most directly to the topic of this study is the research I conducted for my first book, *Cut It Out: The C-Section Epidemic in United States*. For this book, I interviewed physicians, midwives, and nurses about why the U.S. cesarean rate—32 percent in 2016—is so high.[13] What became clear to me in conducting research for *Cut It Out* is how nurses are essential to women's labor and birth experiences.[14] This work led to my fascination with OB nurses, and I could think of no better way to study OB nurses than to spend time with them as they care for patients during labor and delivery, especially during a time of organizational change.[15]

An initial example of how the change and uncertainty faced by Fuller Hospital were front and center during my study was a May 2014 public meeting presented by hospital administrators and potential acquisition partners titled "Preparing for the Future." I describe the meeting below as a way of illustrating the centrality of political, economic, and organizational change at Fuller Hospital.

I arrive in the auditorium about fifteen minutes before the meeting is slated to begin, and the room quickly fills. There is a nervous tension in the air. The CEO of Fuller steps to the microphone. The senior vice president of Axiom and a representative from Elite University are seated behind him on the stage. All three are middle-aged white men dressed in conservative business attire. The CEO of Fuller tells the audience that being acquired by Axiom and Elite University will lead to the best possible future for the hospital.

He continues, telling the audience that the acquisition process began more than two years ago, in December 2011, when the hospital's board studied the landscape and realized that an "asset purchase agreement" was in the hospital's best interest. The CEO tells the audience that Axiom and Elite University have formed a strategic alliance in which Axiom will contribute investment capital and Elite will contribute clinical excellence. He assures the audience that, even with the involvement of an out-of-state corporation like Axiom, health care will continue to be delivered locally. This will create a "sustainable community-based health system."

Axiom, Elite, and Fuller representatives make their case for change. They argue that hospitals are receiving declining reimbursements from the federal government and that this will only get worse with further implementation of the ACA. Therefore, it is necessary for the hospital to find a way to keep costs down to increase equity and to reinvest. Axiom's vice president tells the audience that this is the wave of the future. As an example, he says that equipment that costs Fuller one dollar and Elite University seventy cents costs Axiom only fifty cents. Thus, if costs are to remain low, this is the best solution—to be acquired and to join this strategic alliance. In fact, Fuller's CEO declares that if Fuller Hospital jobs are to be preserved, a partnership is necessary.

Beyond the effects of the ACA, Fuller's CEO argues that the state has changed health-care policy in a way that is hurting the hospital financially. The state instituted a new tax on hospitals that cost Fuller $4.8 million in 2013 and will cost $6.8 million in 2014 and $8.6 million in 2015. The state tax is on top of the 2 percent "sequestration" by the federal government, which costs about $2 million per year. The effect of these policy changes, according to the CEO, is that Fuller has very little money to reinvest in the hospital. In 2013, the reinvestment in the hospital was a mere $100,000. The meeting continues with the hospital and corporate representatives making their case, in turn, over and over again.

Of course, what the representatives are not highlighting is that Fuller, with the acquisition, will transition from a non-profit to a for-profit hospital. However, the audience cannot be duped. The audience's questions and comments are focused on this issue—the community is losing a locally controlled, non-profit, community hospital. There is pushback by community members who see the hospital turning into something it has never been before—a corporation, a for-profit entity, a health provider controlled by out-of-state actors. The audience gives example after example of their good care and their belief that this good care is tied to its being delivered by a community-based, non-profit hospital.

This meeting and impending organizational change are both suggestive of how state and federal policy changes created rapid shifts in the political-economic environment of hospitals. Because these new policies were implemented in a short time frame, I was presented a unique opportunity to study how swift political-economic change affects hospitals and, most important, the human relationships within them. I did this by conducting an interpretive study of the changing nature of interactions, communications, and relationships between nurses and patients in the OB unit of Fuller Hospital, during a particular historical juncture and within a particular organizational context. In the work below I address the following question: How does the process of hospital organizational change in response to sweeping health-care policy shifts affect nurses' relationships with and care of patients?

Existing Research

There is much research on how women are supported during labor and birth, with support examined broadly across several different types of caregivers. Most of this literature examines the benefit of continuous one-on-one support. It is well established by several randomized trials and confirmed in the meta-analyses of these trials that women who have one-on-one support in labor, especially continuous support, experience several benefits over women who do not, including a shorter labor, a lower rate of operative (cesarean) and instrumental (forceps and vacuum) delivery, and a higher level of satisfaction with the birth experience.[16] Women with continuous one-on-one support also are less likely to use intrapartum analgesia or regional analgesia or to have a baby with a low Apgar score at five minutes.[17]

This literature focuses primarily on the continuous support provided by doulas, although a few of the studies examine care given by nurses, midwives, students, volunteers, and/or family members. Research suggests women benefit the most from support that comes from someone outside the hospital staff and outside the woman's social network.[18] A doula is the most likely support person to fit this criterion. Yet, less than 5 percent of women who give birth in the U.S. are supported by a doula.[19]

The literature on nursing support focuses on what they do to support patients, and the key word to notice here is "support." A fairly straightforward definition of support is "to enhance the patient's participation in the labor process and to foster activity which enables the participants to maintain control."[20] Claudia Anderson included in this definition a nurse's promoting the patient's dignity through making sure she is clean, protecting her privacy, and ensuring her comfort.[21] She also included a nurse's providing encouragement and reassurance.[22] Diane Lindo Kintz defined support a bit more broadly to include helping a woman to relax and cope with uterine contractions and manipulating the environment to minimize any distractions.[23] Research also shows that a woman's perception of and ability to cope with pain may be affected by the support of her nurse.[24]

Other scholars focus on how postpartum women look back on and define supportive behavior they experienced during their labors. Robert Klein and colleagues found that postpartum women view nurses as having been supportive when they were present, when they talked to and presented a comfort item to the patient, and when they modeled breathing techniques for the patient.[25] Donna Shields also found in interviews of postpartum women that nurses' having been present is an important element of support, as is teaching and explaining.[26] Further, postpartum women consider a nurse's having offered reassurance, comfort, concern, and conversation to be supportive.[27]

Reducing the cesarean rate (which, as mentioned above, is currently 32 percent) is a popular public health topic.[28] An interesting way of looking at the effect of nursing care on the likelihood of cesarean is by examining how nurses with low cesarean rates provide care differently than do nurses with high rates. The women who are cared for by nurses with low cesarean rates have shorter labors and are less likely to have an instrumental delivery (i.e., forceps and vacuum extraction).[29] Further, how the nurses separated into groups of low- and high-rate cesarean nurses cannot be explained by patient or physician characteristics.[30] This is evidence that the care nurses provide is essential and that not all nurses provide the same type or level of care.

What the research concludes, when viewed holistically, is that women are supported best through one-on-one care that is continuous throughout labor and birth, and that nurses have an important role in women's birth experiences and outcomes. However, the type of care nurses give to patients depends greatly on hospital policies, protocols, and resources, which may limit or encourage supportive nursing care.

Enacting Change

One need not be a social scientist to understand that organizational rules and regulations drive the human behavior within those organizations. We bus our own tables at McDonald's, carry out our own groceries at the supermarket, and stand in line to register our automobiles at the department of motor vehicles. There is no doubt that organizational imperatives drive our behavior. Otherwise, there would not be such similarity in behavior *within* organizations. In short, we live in a society in which most of our time is spent in organizations (e.g., businesses, stores, hospitals, schools, churches, clubs, hospitals), and these organizations direct our behavior.[31]

However, organizations do not exist in a vacuum. Rather, they are situated within a political-economic environment.[32] When the political-economic environment changes, this affects the organization, and the organization proactively responds to changes in the political economy.[33] This is especially the case when organizations face uncertainty, particularly with regard to acquiring needed resources to accomplish organizational goals.[34] In a domino-like effect, when organizations change, the behavior of individuals within the organization must change in response.[35]

In this book I show how top-level administrators focused on state and federal policy changes as a driver that necessitated the financial acquisition of the hospital by another hospital or hospital system. Although policy changes may not be solely responsible for the hospital's response, organizational theory does suggest that the environment of the organization that drives organizational change is "enacted."[36] In other words, organizational administrators interpret what the dependencies are in the environment, to which of these dependencies to react, and what the reaction should be.[37] I suggest that Fuller Hospital executives interpreted state and federal policy changes as problematic, thereby necessitating acquisition, a particular solution. I want to emphasize, however, that it is possible, perhaps even likely, that Fuller executives used the excuse of the ACA and state policy changes to enact changes in the hospital that may not have been legitimized during previous times. Yet, that does not make the effect of policy changes any less real to the hospital's employees and patients.

I integrate a macro-micro linkage by focusing on how organizational changes made by the hospital administrators and board members affected nurses' daily interaction with patients. I argue that nurses are expected to absorb the impact of organizational change—the associated uncertainty and changing resources—through modifying their interactions with and care of patients.[38] Here is one example that the literature misses in terms of what nurses actually do for patients that shows how nurses support patients, and how that support is dependent on nurses' having time to devote to patient care. One of the ways support should be thought of as different than previously explored concerns how nurses help patients negotiate the hospital bureaucracy. This example comes from my first observation at Fuller Hospital in the summer of 2013. Rachel has a patient who has changed her mind about her birth plan after arriving at the hospital. She had scheduled a repeat cesarean, but she reconsiders and wants to attempt a vaginal birth after cesarean (VBAC). The physician on call from the patient's OB group supports her decision but with reservations, as becomes clear. Rachel asks the doctor if it is acceptable to delete the patient's cesarean plan of care on the computer and to submit a vaginal birth plan of care instead. The physician tells her to put the cesarean plan of care "on hold" but not to delete it. "I don't want to jinx her," the physician tells Rachel. Yet, with this plan of care still active in the computer, other departments in the hospital view the patient as a cesarean patient, and the lab sends up a phlebotomist to draw blood for required tests done before surgery. When the phlebotomist arrives at the patient's room to draw the blood, Rachel jumps up from the front desk and asks very pointedly, "Can I help you?" The phlebotomist explains that he has an order to draw blood from the patient. Rachel explains to him that the patient is going to attempt a vaginal birth and, therefore, does not need the blood test. Ever polite, she thanks him for coming up to the unit (a considerable walk). As he leaves, Rachel breathes a sigh of relief and says, "I'm glad I saw him."

My guess is that most women laboring in the hospital would want such a nurse to take care of them. Yet the research that looks at supportive care by nurses would likely have missed such care because of the typical lack of continual focus on a nurses' behavior throughout her shift. Further, I am not confident that Rachel or other nurses would recall this behavior as being a way that they support their patients. In short, researchers *and* nurses have narrow definitions of support that do not capture the complexity of supportive nurse behavior. It is also important to notice that Rachel's preventing an unnecessary blood draw was dependent on her seeing the phlebotomist going to the patient's room, something made possible by her devoting care to only one patient.

Nurse behavior, like that of Rachel in this example, may align with her understanding of the organization's goal being outstanding patient care. Yet the organizational actions and intra-organizational relationships may affect her ability to provide this type of care, and the nurse must mitigate this effect. Such advocacy also requires the nurse to have the time and resources to focus on each patient she is assigned. I classify such nurses as patient oriented. They concern themselves with empathetic care and task themselves with delivering such care, even if the hospital and changes it undergoes make that difficult. I contrast patient-oriented nurses with process-oriented nurses. The latter are also concerned about patient care, but they embrace following hospital rules and protocols as the best way to deliver that care. For example, Julie, a process-oriented nurse, tells me that if patients ask her for care not consistent with hospital protocols, she pulls out the protocol manual and shows the written protocol to them. Process-oriented nurses experience organizational change as making it difficult to meet all the rules and protocols, and this causes them stress. I explore these differences among nurses, the way these differences affect patient care, and, most important, how rapid organizational change affects nurse strategies.

Research Methods

This book is a case study of one hospital unit, Fuller Hospital's OB unit, over a specific time frame, the three-year period of July 2013 through June 2016. A case study is appropriate for this research. As Charles Ragin argues, "The goals of case-oriented investigation often are both historically interpretative and causally analytic. Interpretive work . . . attempts to account for significant historical outcomes . . . by piecing evidence together in a manner sensitive to historical chronology and offering limited historical generalizations which are sensitive to context."[39] Further, according to Ragin, scholars who "use case-oriented strategies often want to understand or interpret specific cases because of their intrinsic value."[40] The key here is to see that this interpretive research examining nurses' experiences, which allows in-depth investigation of one unit within one hospital, has intrinsic value because of how political-economic changes (the ACA and state policies) are affecting it. Further, by conducting a case study, I control for the varied cultures in different sites and the varied politics of different states.[41] This is important because studies have found that hospitals differ greatly on obstetrical outcomes. For example, researchers have found a tenfold variation in hospital cesarean rates.[42] Another study argues that the fact that cesarean rates vary greatly by hospital and geographic region "demonstrates that hospitals and clinicians can differ in their response to the same conditions."[43] Thus, for a case study, an OB unit in a single hospital is the perfect laboratory for examining how rapid and sweeping health-care policy change affects nurses and nurse-patient interactions.[44]

I use two types of data to study this hospital and explore how OB nurses are affected by organizational change in response to shifts in the political economy. First, I conducted ethnographic observations of obstetrical nurses at Fuller Hospital. I shadowed nineteen nurses for a total of 233 hours between July 2013 and June 2016. Second, I conducted in-depth interviews with twenty-one obstetrical nurses and four unit administrators to further my understanding of how the role of nurses has changed in the wake of the ACA and state-level policy changes as well as organizational changes happening in the hospital. I both followed and interviewed fourteen nurses. I gave all nurses and administrators pseudonyms, and I categorize nurses' years of experience rather than giving the exact number of years of experience to prevent deductive disclosure of their identities to other research participants or employees of Fuller Hospital.

To understand how I carried out this research, I start with information about how I picked Fuller Hospital to study, how I gained access to the OB unit, and how I conducted the observations and interviews. I feel it important to discuss these issues because birth is very much affected by the hospital in which the birth takes place. Yet hospitals as places are not, per se, actors. Rather, the employees of hospitals—administrators, nurses, physicians, staff—are what make hospitals different from one another. Further, as pointed out by Gary Fine and David Shulman, it is important for ethnographers to share the nitty-gritty detail of the study, less it seem glossed over and not reflective of what actually happens in the organization.[45]

I was fortunate to find a community hospital near my home—Fuller—where I was welcomed into the OB unit. This hospital is in a New England metropolitan area with a population of one million. It is physically part of a surrounding suburb with a population of just over fifty thousand. In 2013, the hospital oversaw around 1,200 births per year. Two practices that include multiple physicians and midwives—one practice with one obstetrician and one midwife, and one solo obstetrician practice—had privileges at Fuller Hospital when I began my study in 2013. In March 2015, the hospital added two more practices—one that has four obstetricians and one midwife, and one that has two midwives—and births increased by 25 percent, to about 1,500 per year.

My access to the hospital was built on a request I made to the nurse manager of the unit in 2012 for my undergraduate students in a class on the sociology of reproduction I taught at a nearby college to complete a service-learning placement in the unit. The students in this class were required to volunteer twenty hours over the course of the semester in an organization that somehow dealt with reproduction. Many students typically volunteered in a tertiary-care hospital near the college. But Fuller Hospital, about a twenty-minute drive from the school, was quite different from the other hospital, and I wanted students to have an opportunity to volunteer at a community hospital that, at the time, had about half as many births per year as the tertiary care hospital. Fuller Hospital also had some of the best perinatal measures in the state. The nurse manager agreed to have two students volunteer. However, much to my chagrin, I could not persuade any of the students to make the drive to this hospital for their service-learning requirement.

Even though my students did not volunteer at this hospital, I became intrigued with the idea of studying it. The hospital had key characteristics that attracted my interest. First, it had one of the lowest cesarean rates in the state. Second, several doulas (birth assistants) I knew told me it was the "best" hospital in the state in which to give birth. Third, it was close to my home, making the study easy to conduct.

The positive interaction I had previously with the nurse manager, although limited, allowed me to get my foot in the door. I contacted the nurse manager by email and asked about conducting a study in the unit. She was both supportive and enthusiastic, and directed me to Nancy, the OB clinical nursing education specialist, who was just as, if not more, enthusiastic about the study.[46] The nurse manager also connected me to the hospital's institutional review board (IRB) director. I applied for and received approval from the IRB at both the hospital and the college by which I was employed, and, once I had done so, I set up a meeting with the OB clinical nursing education specialist.[47]

We agree to meet on a lovely summer day in 2013. I drive to the hospital, a bundle of nervous energy and excitement. I park my car in the parking lot closest to the unit and walk uphill to the entrance, which has a circle drive in front where valet staff wait for cars to park, a free service to patients. The valet staff greet me with a friendly hello, something they almost invariably did each time I came to the hospital. There is a center revolving door and a single traditional glass door entrance to the building. I almost always followed the posted request to use the revolving door. The door opens onto a reception desk for another hospital unit. The receptionist sits behind a sliding window about eight feet from the entrance. Sometimes the receptionist noticed me and said hello, but typically I walked by unnoticed. Immediately to the left are stairs, and immediately to the right is an elevator. The OB unit is on the third floor of the building. I choose the stairs (my students will tell you that "get your steps in" is one of my mantras) and proceed up to the third floor. The stairwell is unkempt, rather dirty, and seldom used. The metal banister and rails are painted turquoise, and on the landing between the second and third floors there is a dated, framed print of fluffy white flowers in a vase next to a glass bowl filled with peaches. Coming on to the unit from the stairs, a quick left turn places me in front of Nancy's office, where she warmly greets me before escorting me to the education room, catty-corner from her office.

My meeting with Nancy is positive and productive. I learn that she is supportive of my research, especially my focus on nurses. We connect over our shared passion for women's health issues. She tells me about herself and how she ended up in her current position. Her journey involved hard work, heartbreak, the importance of family, and an ever-present passion for women's health. Nancy gives me a tour of the unit, introducing me to nurses and staff alike along the way. She takes me into a "ready room," to show me a typical LDRP (labor, delivery, recovery, and postpartum) room, and into one of the triage rooms as well. She also shows me one of the larger, extended-stay rooms, where women recover following cesareans.

At the end of the tour, Nancy tells me that the hospital is going to partner with another hospital or hospital system because it is facing severe financial problems. She tells me that a "partner" has not yet been chosen. She expresses a guarded optimism but also makes clear the uncertainty faced by hospital administrators and staff. It is at this moment that I know I am in the perfect place because I am given the opportunity to study nurses *during organizational change.* We end the visit amicably, and I promise to email Nancy next week, when I plan to start observations.

Nancy serves as my guide once again the following week when I come to the hospital to observe the nurses for the first time. I share an excerpt from my observational note to set the scene:

> I arrived in the unit at 7:45 a.m. Nancy had asked me to find her in the education room where we met before. She was teaching a class for new nurses, but would tell them that she would need to leave to introduce me around. I found the room, right off the elevator. Nancy immediately jumped up and told the students that they had a fifteen-minute break. She seemed very glad to see me. . . . I have noticed in both of my visits that she seems very busy, and she had told me that she has a number of responsibilities.

Nancy uses the fifteen-minute break to escort me around the unit. I ask her where I can stow my purse, and she shows me the counter in the break room, already littered with purses and bags. She tells me that everyone leaves their purses there, although the room is not locked. She then takes me around the unit and introduces me around, attempting to find a nurse for me to shadow. Again, I draw on my notes:

> I told Nancy I had brought bakery cookies for the nurses and placed them on the break table. The nurses present seemed very appreciative of the cookies. Nancy then introduced me to everyone at the table. . . . She seemed unsure how to explain my research [but did] introduce me as a professor of sociology. . . . Nancy asked them if there were many patients, and we heard about a woman scheduled for a repeat c-section who now wanted to VBAC. Nancy then walked me to the main desk and introduced me to . . . the secretary and . . . the charge nurse. She asked [the charge nurse] if there was a labor patient.

It is in this interaction that Nancy's support of my research becomes clear; when the charge nurse hesitates at Nancy's request for a nurse for me to shadow, Nancy follows by asking, "What about the surprise VBAC patient?" The charge nurse, rather unenthusiastically, says that

Rachel has the patient and that I can ask her if it is okay for me to follow her. Nancy takes me to find Rachel, who seems excited to be involved in the research. Rachel tells me that her patient is walking, but that on her next round (the unit is configured in a square shape) she'll have her go to her room for monitoring and will ask her then if it would be ok for me to follow her. I sit at the desk and wait. At this point, Nancy leaves me to Rachel and returns to her class. Rachel returns soon after to tell me the patient is happy to have me observe. I was fortunate to have Nancy as a supporter because she eased my way into finding the first nurse to observe, which would likely have been more of a challenge on my own.

I received consent from nurses and patients to observe them. The way informed consent for nurses and patients worked is that I asked the nurse for permission to follow and interview her. I went over the consent form with each nurse and asked her to sign the form. I gave an extra copy of the form to the nurse to keep. All nurses I followed and/or interviewed signed these forms. Then, the nurse approached her patient without me to ask for permission for me to observe her care. If the patient agreed, and almost all did, I entered the room and discussed the study with the patient. I gave each patient an information sheet with facts about the study and her rights as a participant. I also went over the sheet with the patient and left it with her. All IRBs involved allowed me to waive documentation of the patients' consent so that I would not have to collect their names. Collecting patient names would link patients to the study and, in that way, increase their risk of participating. In short, not collecting names meant that there is no way patients could be identified in any research publications. All IRBs preferred waiving documentation of consent to my collecting patient names.

In terms of my observations, I followed nurses in all their activities, including their time spent in patient care and documentation but also in the more social times of breakfast, lunch, coffee breaks, and, occasionally, smoking breaks. I interacted with many more nurses than I followed, and I also interacted with physicians and midwives during my time at the hospital. I draw on these experiences as well. My hours of observations allowed me to develop an understanding of what nurses do in their day-to-day work life and, especially, how organizational change affects them.

I sometimes talked with patients, but typically only when they initiated conversation. I met some interesting people. My most memorable interaction was when I introduced myself to a patient and her doula said excitedly, "You're Theresa Morris? I'm reading your book [*Cut It Out: The C-Section Epidemic in America*]! I can't believe I'm meeting you!" I call this interaction my "five seconds of fame." Other interesting people include a couple, both music teachers who played the same, somewhat obscure instrument. With a few questions and encouragement from the nurse, they told us their courtship story, which involved a failed blind date and then a chance meeting at a music teachers' conference. This meeting led to a successful date and ultimately serious relationship. Another interesting experience was when a patient's mother-in-law repeatedly showed the nurse and me videos of her dog. She had narrated the videos as though the dog were talking. Some patients and their families and/or friends asked me questions about my research, but most did not. I was always struck with how open patients and their families were in allowing me to observe as they went through such a meaningful and intimate experience.

In terms of interviews, I conducted them with nurses in the break room, in empty "ready" rooms, and over the phone. I sometimes interviewed nurses one-on-one, and I sometimes interviewed nurses in pairs or groups. I asked nurses questions about how they care for patients and about the effects of changes in the hospital on them and on their care of patients.

Plan for the Book

The first part of the book introduces the hospital, OB unit, and what nurses do. Chapter 1 lays out the hospital and OB unit in which I conducted observations. I paint a picture of the hospital—its location, physical structure, and culture. In Chapter 2, I detail the roles of OB nurses, including their responsibilities and common tasks. This chapter, chock-full of the details of what an OB nurse does, ends with an overview of how changes affected the OB nurses at Fuller Hospital.

The second part of the book is the heart of the analysis and focuses on how nurses have dealt with changes at the hospital. By examining nurses' experience and interaction with patients, it becomes possible to compare how the same organizational change affects nurses differently. In the end, all nurses must adapt, and this adaptation trickles down to how patients experience care. I structure the chapters by focusing on specific nurses, my observations and interviews with them before Axiom pulled its acquisition offer in December 2014 (pre-Axiom) and my observations and interviews with them after Axiom pulled out (post-Axiom). I use the Axiom acquisition collapse as a distinguishing point because it was this event that sent the hospital, already under financial constraints, into a tailspin.

Chapter 3 features nurses whose primary focus is on patient care. Because of this, patients love to have them as their nurses. Patient-oriented nurses have different backgrounds and years of experience but have in common spending long periods of time with patients. When they are not in the patient's room, they are finding ways to advocate for the patient out of the room or to advocate for other patients or for programs they believe are important. These nurses respond to organizational change by attempting to buffer patients from any negative effects, which causes the nurses much frustration and stress, and they are not always successful in their attempts to buffer patients.

In Chapter 4, I examine nurses I define as process oriented. They spend less time with patients and focus their care on following rules and protocols dictated by the hospital. These nurses, like patient-oriented nurses, are different in terms of background and years of experience. But, different from patient-oriented nurses, process-oriented nurses are in and out of the room as quickly as possible, with more time spent sitting at the desk documenting. These nurses are affected by organizational changes, but not in the same way as patient-oriented nurses because they do not spend as much time with patients. Their experience has more to do with learning new protocols and routines and managing the documentation of an increased patient load.

The third part of the book focuses on the political-economic and organizational changes that affected the nurses. The political economy of this hospital has transformed at both the national and state level, and these changes have resulted in organizational change. Chapter 5 situates the human relationships involved in giving birth in hospitals within the historical and institutional contexts of 2013–16. This chapter lays out the national policy change—the ACA—and state-level policy changes and suggests how they had clear effects on this hospital.

In the book's conclusion, I reflect on the book's findings and on how this study of nurses of Fuller Hospital is an example of how political-economic changes and organizational decisions about how to respond to those changes affect nurses and patient care. I include in the conclusion a public sociology discussion of how the book's findings can inform how nurses advocate for change and how women choose a place to give birth.

Conclusion

I end the chapter by declaring my support of the Affordable Care Act. It is my hope that readers will remember this as they read the book and its critique of what I argue are consequences of the ACA. The ACA undertakes needed reforms to U.S. health care to insure more people and solves the uncertainty of insurance coverage for many people and many procedures. This book should not be seen primarily as a critique of the ACA, but as a nuanced examination of how consequences of the ACA (and hospitals' responses to them) may put small community hospitals and their employees and patients at risk.

PART I

Fuller Hospital

1

Welcome to the Obstetric Unit

In order for me to take care of my patients, I need to be . . . in the room, helping them [with] whatever they need . . . You're a breastfeeding mom, and you need help breastfeeding, I should be able to be in the room with you for a significant period of time. But, with no staff and high priorities walking in the door, the people who get left behind are all the others—the people who aren't an emergency. So, you're triaging and prioritizing who's going to get taken care of because you don't have anyone to take care of all the people. So, that's pretty much what we're functioning under every single night. "Oh yeah, that's great. You need breastfeeding help, but this one's bleeding to death. So, you're not going to get breastfeeding help because I need to take her to the operating room." So, every single night that's how I feel when I go to work. (Jamie)

Jamie is indicting change that is significant. Fuller Hospital used to be "the place to give birth." It had a reputation within the community and local area for respecting women's wishes, especially if the woman had very specific ideas about how she wanted to give birth. I found that this assessment was consistent with the nurses' feeling that Fuller hospital was also a "good" place to work—at least this was the general feeling of nurses when I started the study in July 2013. At the beginning of my study, I found the OB nurses, in general, really enjoyed working at the hospital, and several nurses commuted a considerable distance to work there, even though they lived closer to other hospitals. Nurses expressed satisfaction that physicians and midwives valued and respected them and gave them considerable autonomy. However, by the time my study ended three years later, many nurses, like Jamie, felt that change at the hospital had not been kind to them, and they were not as satisfied or happy with their jobs. Although they still felt valued by the midwives and physicians, they felt downtrodden by administrative decisions that left the unit busier, understaffed, and perpetually full beyond capacity.

This chapter sets the stage for the coming chapters with an understanding of Fuller Hospital and its OB unit as a place.

Fuller Hospital, Then and Now

I start with a brief overview of the history of Fuller Hospital to make the point that it is a *community* hospital, founded for a community need with community resources. Thus, its being acquired by an out-of-state, for-profit hospital is a drastic change. Nearly one hundred years old, Fuller dates back to the 1918 Spanish influenza pandemic that killed as many as fifty million people worldwide.[1] Although the hospital had not been established yet when the pandemic struck, the community opened a temporary emergency hospital in a local hall to deal with the sick. This pandemic spurred a campaign to open a permanent hospital in Fuller. The community kicked off a campaign that raised $165,000 ($2.3 million in 2017 dollars) in less than a week, leading to the construction of the hospital, which opened in 1920.[2] The hospital was dedicated to men from Fuller who died in World War I.

Fast-forward to 1961, when Fuller Hospital opened one of the first community hospital birthing rooms in the United States. At that time, it was also one of the first U.S. hospitals to offer the Lamaze method of childbirth. In line with its emphasis on women's health, in 1993 Fuller Hospital opened a family support and resource center, which offers parent programs and family support services.[3]

Although Fuller began as an independent hospital, it joined forces with another community hospital, Marple, in 1995 when the corporators of the two hospitals voted to merge corporate parents and form Directional Health Network (DHN). The merger was approved by the state in 1995 and was noted as an unusual merger because both Fuller and Marple were financially sound. Following the merger, both hospitals remained fully intact and operated independently. Over the next ten years, Fuller Hospital expanded, sometimes by partnering with other hospitals, to open a regional radiation therapy service for cancer treatment, wellness center, sleep disorders laboratory, and comprehensive cancer care center.[4]

In 2004, Fuller Hospital opened the Family Birth Center, "offering state-of-the-art LDRP rooms and an enhanced level of service."[5] Just six years later, Marple Hospital ended its childbirth services, sending women who receive prenatal and postnatal care at the hospital's clinic to give birth at Fuller Hospital.[6] Fuller's absorption of Marple's patients is still somewhat contentious for two reasons. First, several OB nurses moved from Marple to Fuller when Marple's unit closed, and they lost their seniority for such things as signing up for vacation days. Second, Marple's patients now come to Fuller to deliver, and many of them are "clinic" patients (Marple still has a clinic that sees mostly patients who lack private health insurance). These uninsured patients are often ridiculed and, at least socially, treated differently by many nurses and physicians. The two largest OB practices that deliver at Fuller share responsibility for the care of Marple's "clinic" patients, but neither of the practices is happy with this arrangement. The family practice residents are supposed to oversee these patients' care, but that rarely happens, sometimes because the nurses cannot get a hold of the residents or do not try, seeing them as unqualified because they are not OB residents but rather family medicine residents.

In 2015, Fuller Hospital employed roughly 1,135 full-time employees and maintained 181 beds. The hospital's occupancy rate hovered in the 70 percent range from 2011 to 2014, dropping to 62 percent in 2015, a significant decline from the upper 80 percent range from 2006 to 2010, although this is at least partly a result of adding more beds. There were 29,106 emergency visits in 2006 and 44,832 in 2007. The number of such visits increased gradually over the next six years to 47,065 in 2013 before dropping to 39,779 in 2015.[7]

Fuller Hospital's percentage of Medicaid patients has increased 20 percent since 2011, likely a result of the spread of Medicaid coverage in the state. In terms of payer mix for charges, in 2015, 22 percent of hospital charges were *incurred* by Medicaid, and 16.2 percent were *paid* by Medicaid. These percentages are slightly higher than state averages, which had 21.4 percent of hospital charges *incurred* by Medicaid and 12.5 percent *paid* by Medicaid in 2015. The difference between Medicaid charges incurred and paid is due to Medicaid's paying hospitals in the state, for example, in 2014 on average 63 cents for every dollar of incurred costs.[8]

A common financial measure indicating the health of hospitals is margin, calculated as income from operations divided by total operating revenues, which is then multiplied by one hundred. In 2013, Fuller Hospital had a negative margin, for the first time since 2006. In 2015, the margin rose to 3.9 percent, still well below the 5.22 percent level of 2008 and the 5 percent level of 2012.[9] Further, According to data compiled by the state Office of Health Care Access, in fiscal year 2015 Fuller Hospital had a ratio (dollars of current assets per dollar of current liabilities) of 1.19, well below the state average of 2.15, and a lower number of days of cash on hand—eleven days compared to the state average of seventy-eight days.[10]

Due to the financial struggles it was facing, in 2010 Fuller began to explore the option of being acquired by another hospital or hospital system. As mentioned in the prior chapter, there was a failed acquisition attempt in 2015 before Fuller was successfully acquired by a for-profit hospital system, Waranoke Heath System, on October 1, 2016.

In the years between when acquisition was sought and accomplished, the hospital introduced various initiatives to shore up its finances. Two of these had direct impacts on the OB unit. First, In July 2013, the hospital added a residency program, and the residents rotate through the OB unit. Second, in March 2015, two new OB practices affiliated with the OB unit at Fuller, increasing the number of births at the hospital by 25 percent.

The Obstetric Unit at Fuller Hospital

The OB unit at Fuller Hospital is what is referred to as an LDRP, or a labor, delivery, recovery, and postpartum unit. When a woman is admitted as a patient to the unit, she is assigned a room in which she will labor, deliver, recover, and (often) stay after the baby is born until she, and usually the baby, is discharged. This is one of only a few LDRP units in the state, and some women come to the hospital to give birth specifically for an LDRP-unit experience. In such a unit, nurses are trained to take care of both laboring and postpartum patients.[11] Many hospitals separate the labor and delivery unit from the postpartum unit. In such hospitals, nurses specialize in either labor and delivery or postpartum care and obstetrical patients transition from one unit and set of nurses (labor and delivery) to an entirely different unit and set of nurses (postpartum) during a typical hospital stay for the birth of a baby. The OB

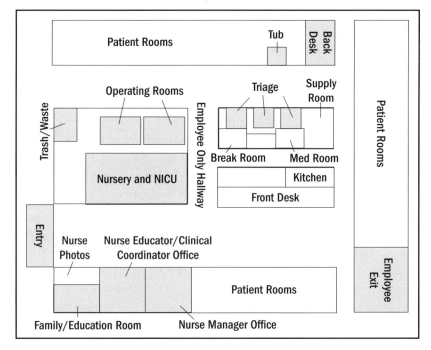

Figure 1.1. Layout of the obstetric unit in Fuller Hospital.

unit also has dedicated NICU (neonatal intensive care unit) nurses. Most OB nurses do not work in the NICU, although a few do have the credentials and training to float into the NICU when the NICU is busy.

Figure 1.1 presents a rough diagram—not to exact scale—of the OB unit at Fuller Hospital. I have identified specific features, such as nurse desks, the break room, the operating rooms, and offices, in dark gray. The entry—which requires a hospital-issued ID to open or someone at the desk (typically a secretary or nurse) to buzz a visitor in—opens onto the front hall. There is a parallel long hall in the back of the unit. As one walks into the unit, photos of the unit's nurses are displayed on the right, although the photos have not been updated in some time. The offices for the nurse manager of the unit and a shared office for the OB clinical nursing education specialist and clinical coordinator are found on the right, past these photos. The education specialist and clinical coordinator used to share an office that was just outside the unit, and the office they now occupy on the unit was used by the NICU physicians and advanced practitioners. However, at the request of the NICU doctors and staff, these office functions were flipped in late 2015. Across the hall from that office are the nursery and NICU. The education room, where different educational programs and staff meetings and events are held, is only accessible from an entrance outside the unit. Its doorway is next to the entryway door to the unit.

The two areas where nurses congregate most are the front desk, which is open to the hallway and in front of patient rooms, and the break room, which is located off the employee-only hall. The front desk is where nurses sit when they care for patients but are out of the room or have not yet been assigned a patient. Nurses sit behind a counter, on which sits, facing outward, a sculpture of a man, woman, and two babies (a plaque indicates that it is a gift from a local obstetrician) and a sculpture of a woman holding a baby. The counter also displays a variety of informational pamphlets for patients, although I never witnessed a patient looking at or taking one. On the other side of the counter and at a much lower height is a long, built-in counter-like desk, which houses two computers, each with two monitors, for the nurses; one computer for the midwives and physicians; one computer for the secretary, who sits at the far side of the desk, closest to the entry door; and one computer that shows the rooms and, when a patient presses the call button, indicates from what room the call is coming. The desk is typically littered with coffee cups—ceramic, paper, plastic, and Styrofoam—as well as soda and seltzer cans and bottles. The office chairs at this desk face the counter. Often the chairs have discarded scrub jackets or sweatshirts adorning their backs. Patients and family members often come to this counter to ask questions or make requests. Above the desk and to the right is a television screen hung from the ceiling, which displays the image of anyone calling to be let into the unit as well as images of the unit hallways.

Besides sitting at the desk, the nurses also stand and lean against or sit on a counter about three feet behind the desk. This is where the protocol binder is kept, as are various devices, such as a tool to help one learn how to measure cervical dilation and a wheel to date a woman's pregnancy, a sign-up sheet to have a lactation consultant visit a patient, other manuals and binders (e.g., staff meeting minutes, secretary how-to manual, OR terminal cleaning manual, patient callback binder, order supply binder, front desk phone book), and glucose monitoring kits.

Above the back counter are three full-sized cabinets, which hold various office supplies, and two half-sized cabinets with vertical cubbies below them in which patient files are stored by room number.

Some notices are hung on the wall underneath the cabinets, the most interesting of which I found to be a chart that identifies which oversight organization—the Department of Public Health (DPH), the Joint Commission (TJC), the Centers for Medicare and Medicaid Services (CMS), or the insurance carrier—must be notified in the case of specific adverse events, such as patient death due to medication error or infant discharged to wrong person (DPH), unanticipated death of a full-term infant (TJC), death while in restraint or seclusion (CMS), or any unexpected death (insurance carrier). This process always involves notifying the hospital's risk management department, evidence of what I have found in other research to be a heavy focus of hospitals on liability in obstetrics.[12] In fact, more arrows on the chart point to the risk management department and to the hospital counsel than to the quality improvement department, a rather stunning observation.[13]

Nurses use the computers at the desk to monitor the electronic "strip" that displays the fetal heart rate pattern and the woman's contraction pattern, both of which appear on the screen, and to document this information on the patient's electronic medical record. Nurses can also see on the screen an electronic board that looks like a spreadsheet. The rows display all patient rooms in the unit, and the columns show the patient's name, if she has delivered and when, the group practice name, gravidity (number of pregnancies), parity (number of births), and the state of the patient's amniotic sac (intact, ruptured spontaneously, ruptured artificially). The color of the rows designates whether the patient is a laboring patient (salmon), a VBAC patient (magenta), a woman who has a cesarean scheduled (lilac), a postpartum patient who delivered vaginally (aqua), a postpartum patient who delivered by cesarean (purple), a patient being observed (yellow), or an antepartum patient (i.e., a patient who is pregnant and experiencing problems during pregnancy) (green). This color coding allows doctors, midwives, and nurses to quickly look at the screen and get a quick snapshot of the patient mix in the unit.

Besides charting, nurses also use the computers to complete required online training modules, send and receive work emails, and check on work-related issues such as vacation days and pay. Nurses use the phones at the front desk to call physicians and midwives, other nurses, the lab, anesthesiology, pediatricians, the pharmacy, engineering (for any equipment or facility repairs), and IT. They also use the computer and their phones for personal communication, shopping, watching videos, and, sometimes, playing games, although, using work time for personal tasks is technically prohibited. There is even a sign posted near the front desk and back desk with a photo of an old-style flip phone indicating that phones should only be used for patient care. Nurses, physicians, and staff routinely ignore this sign. Nurses' use of cell phones at the desk sometimes causes contention. One nurse lamented to me that some nurses surf the internet, play games on their phones, and chitchat while other nurses "are just working their butts off."

Midwives and physicians congregate at the front desk, too, and there is interaction among and between nurses, midwives, physicians, pediatricians, social workers, and other staff—formal (about patients, charts, etc.) and informal (about family; vacations; doctors, nurses, and patients; gossip, etc.)—such that the noise level is sometimes high. Note that I listed patients as subjects of both formal and informal communication. This is because patients are not only discussed as patients but are also sometimes discussed in a way that I would not deem "official." They are made fun of ("I hate my patient!"; "I can't say my patients name"— followed by a very poor pronunciation of a "foreign" name) or admired ("My patient is so sweet"). Yet, the gossip addresses not only patients but also nurses and physicians. One day one of the nurses was assigned a patient with Asperger's syndrome and was reading about the autism-spectrum disorder when a group of nurses decided that the symptoms described one of the OB nurses who worked on a different shift. Except, one of the nurses says, "she doesn't have that," pointing on the screen to the characteristic "has special talent or skill." They all laugh. I wrote in my notes that their behavior "breaks my heart a little bit." This type of behavior—ridiculing and making fun of other nurses, physicians, and patients—is endemic to the unit. I was struck by how such behavior often took place at the front desk, where patients and their friends and family could overhear.

The noise level behind the front desk sometimes reaches such a high level that patients complain, especially those whose rooms are located near the desk; to deal with these complaints, the administration hung a large plastic ear on the wall behind the desk.[14] The plastic ear turns red when noise at the desk is too loud. This warns those at the desk to quiet down. This ear was taken down toward the end of my observations, but new rules were instituted to try to keep noise down, such as not discussing patients at the front desk. Still, noise was often a problem. I only rarely saw much concern from nurses, midwives, or physicians about the noise level. Further, talk about patients at the front desk continued unabated.

The other place nurses congregate is in the break room. Tucked away on a side hall, the break room is about eight by twelve feet. There is a counter that runs across the long side of the room, which is directly across from the doorway, whose door is always kept open. Nurses put their handbags on this counter. There is a refrigerator, microwave, sink, and coffee maker on the shorter end of the room. Photos from parties, featuring several nurses posing for the camera, are attached to the front of the refrigerator. Nurses typically eat breakfast, lunch, dinner, and snacks in the break room, where there is a large rectangular table and chairs in the center of the room, although if the unit is busy nurses may eat at the front desk. Nurses often leave snacks and treats to share with other nurses on the table in the break room, and sometimes patients bring treats for the nurses, which are also shared on the table in the break room. Most nurses use the refrigerator in the break room to store food, but other nurses walk to the hospital cafeteria to buy food. Doctors and midwives also typically eat their meals in the break room. Although socializing now and then takes place at the front desk, the break room is all about socializing. This is the back stage of the unit, where stories are told, laughter is common, and nurses show their camaraderie most easily. Nurses who have worked at other hospitals or other units of Fuller comment on the rapport among nurses, midwives, and physicians in the OB unit as something unique. I once overhead a nurse and a physician making plans to go holiday shopping together on the weekend.

The break room is also the central work-schedule hub. There is a long bulletin board on the wall adjacent to the door that holds sign-up sheets for required call (OB nurses are required to sign up for twelve hours each month in which they may be called in to work) and vacation, notices about meetings and mandatory training, and nurse requests for someone to cover a shift she is scheduled for but does not want to or cannot work. Patient satisfaction survey data for the unit are also displayed on this board. If comments mention a nurse by name and are positive, administrators leave her name in the comments. If comments mention a nurse by name and are negative, administrators remove her name, although administrators will privately talk to her about the comment. A three-ring binder with schedules typically hangs from a tack on the bulletin board. Available shifts are posted on the door of the break room. These are shifts that need to be filled and for which any nurse on the unit can sign up. Above the counter on the opposite side of the room is a bulletin board labeled "Fun Stuff," which is used to display thank-you and holiday cards and photos, usually of babies, from staff and former patients.

Besides the break room and front desk, nurses sometimes sit at the back desk. This is a much smaller and isolated space and does not face patient rooms like the front desk does. Nurses typically go to the back desk, where there are two computers and three office chairs, to find a quiet place to work on required patient documentation. Or, sometimes, this becomes the home base if a nurse is assigned a patient whose room is on the back hall.

The unit has two fully equipped operating rooms (ORs), used almost exclusively for cesareans. The only other uses, which happened rarely during my observations, are, first, when physicians attempt to perform an external cephalic version (ECV or version) to turn a fetus presenting in a breech position to a head-down position, and, second, when women attempt vaginal delivery of twins. Gynecological surgeries are done in the OR on the first floor of the hospital. The door leading to the ORs is locked. There is a narrow hall between the two ORs where the doors into each are located on opposite sides. Sterile head and shoe coverings, which must be worn in the OR, are also available in the hall. At least one OR is supposed to be set up and ready to go always. This is important in the case of an emergency cesarean. I was in the hospital a few times when it was so busy that neither OR was ready to go, which was a source of stress for the nurses.

The nurses go to the medication room to retrieve all medication, from Tylenol to Percocet to Pitocin, and to the supply room to obtain supplies, from sheets to diapers to lubricant. The supply room has nearly ceiling-high moveable shelving units on wheels, which can be pushed back and forth so that the nurses can gain access to different rows. Sometimes nurses know just where to find a certain supply, and sometimes they do not and must spend time looking. The waste/trash room is located on the back hall. This is where nurses take trash, dirty linens, and dirty equipment.

The unit has three triage rooms and one tub room, all located on the back hall. Nearly all patients are evaluated in a triage room, apart from patients who arrive at the unit clearly in active labor. Such patients are typically placed directly in an LDRP room. If a patient comes to the hospital because she believes she is in labor but is not clearly in labor (a more common occurrence), she is placed in a triage room. Most patients who suspect they are in labor come to the hospital after talking with or seeing their physicians or midwives, although some come without that conversation and a few patients arrive by ambulance. If labor is suspected, nurses evaluate women for telltale signs, and the patient may be kept as an outpatient to "rule out" labor. Such patients are monitored so that nurses can look for a consistent contraction pattern and assess the fetal heartbeat for fetal health. The nurse, physician, or midwife may also check the patient's cervical dilation. If the patient believes her amniotic sac has ruptured, the nurse, midwife, or physician conducts a simple test to see if the patient has amniotic fluid in her vagina, a sign that the sac has ruptured.

What happens next depends on the gestational age of the fetus. For term infants (at least thirty-seven weeks' gestation), if the patient has a ruptured amniotic sac she will be admitted as a patient, given an LDRP room, and assigned a nurse. If her uterus has not started contracting, her provider will almost always induce the patient's labor. If the patient is term and has an intact amniotic sac and the nurse, physician, and/or midwife believes labor may be starting, he or she may ask the patient to walk around the unit for a time to see if the patient's contractions pick up and her cervix changes (i.e., become thinner and/or more dilated). After she walks for a while, a decision is made. If the woman is not found to be in labor, she will typically be sent home. If the patient's cervix has changed and/or her contraction pattern is regular, she will typically be admitted as a patient and assigned an LDRP room and a nurse.

This all changes for pre-term infants (less than thirty-seven weeks' gestation). The course of action depends on how pre-term the infant is, whether the physician or midwife believes labor has actually started, and if so, if labor can be stalled, whether the amniotic sac has ruptured, and whether the infant or woman is ill or has a condition that may influence the doctor and/or midwife's decision about how the patient should be treated and whether the patient will be admitted to the OB unit.

Triage rooms are also used for pregnant patients who display various minor conditions (like a urinary tract infection), have fallen, or are suffering a minor injury or illness. Sometimes nurses are frustrated that doctors (and sometimes midwives) send pregnant patients to the unit who are not in labor but are experiencing a different medical issue. Nurses feel strongly that the OB unit is not appropriate for such patients and that the physician or midwife should see such a patient in an office visit. The nurses get particularly frustrated when such patients arrive in the late afternoon, when physicians' offices are getting ready to close, because they feel the physicians do not want to stay late and, instead, send the patients to the hospital. For more serious medical issues, nurses feel that such patients should be seen in a different unit that deals with the specific medical issue they are facing.

The unit has one tub room for women to use in labor and/or birth. There used to be two tub rooms, but in 2015 one was converted into a third triage room. This change was made to help the unit deal with the increased patient load from the new practices. According to administrator Cynthia, "Now [one of the tub rooms] is a triage room. And, so, we have three of those [triage rooms] now, which makes it a little bit easier to get people through triage." Women may labor in the tub room and, if the physician or midwife allows, have a water birth in which the baby is born while the woman is in the tub. However, in all my observations, I only saw two women use a tub room, and I never was in the hospital when a baby was born in the tub.

Finally, there is a small kitchen for patients to use and for nurses to use in their care of patients. The kitchen has a full-size refrigerator, ice machine (which was broken for a period of time and temporarily replaced with a barrel-like container—like those seen at fairs and in airports—that was filled with ice and sat in the hall outside the kitchen, leading to many jokes by the nurses), and a coffee pot. The nurses go to this kitchen to retrieve water, ice chips, juice, straws, popsicles, and ginger ale for patients. The kitchen is also stocked with crackers (saltine and graham), peanut butter, jelly, Nutri-Grain bars, cocoa, coffee, tea, sugar, and Sweet'N Low for a patient's family and friends. Nurses often, but not always, tell these family and friends that they may go to this kitchen to get snacks and/or beverages or to store food in the refrigerator. Sometimes, when the break-room refrigerator gets full, nurses store their own lunches in the refrigerator in the patient kitchen. Nurses also sometimes snack on food from the kitchen, especially peanut butter.

Conclusion

The key to understanding the recent changes at Fuller Hospital is that most of the funding for the initial building and for its renovations throughout the years has come from the local community. The community prides itself on this hospital, which it sees as part of its identity. Thus, when the political-environment erupts in fast-paced change and the hospital reels financially, it is important to contextualize the response of the hospital with this knowledge. This chapter also contextualizes the physical space of the OB unit, to give the reader a sense of the hospital environment.

2

A Day in the Life of an Obstetrical Nurse

> We run our own triage, which is basically our own emergency room. We run our own OR, so you have to be an OR nurse, too. . . . You have to walk in a room with a screaming patient and be able to calm her down and control things, and you have to stand up to doctors sometimes, and you might have to deliver a baby. That can be scary. You have to [be able to] resuscitate a baby. (Jennifer)

What are the roles of an OB nurse and what policies and rules structure her work life? Jennifer's interview excerpt, above, gives the reader a sense of the demands placed on OB nurses, which may not be appreciated by most, even nurses in other specialties. It is a common frustration of OB nurses that they believe others think they rock babies all day long, which is a very small part of their jobs and something they do not do most days. Lauren, a nurse in the unit, said this in another way by focusing on the different roles of OB nurses:

> I'm a [labor and delivery] nurse. I am a postpartum nurse. I'm a circulating nurse in the OR, and I am a nurse that can scrub in . . . in the OR. . . . The only other thing that I could add under my belt would be to work in the nursery, and I haven't been trained to work in the nursery. . . . Another responsibility, to make it six, is, you know, a lot of our nurses are also charge.

In short, being an OB nurse is a multifaceted job. As Julie succinctly states, "Labor and delivery's not all, 'Oh let's come and have a baby, everything's peachy.' It's not like that." This chapter discusses the typical day of an OB nurse and ends with a discussion of how that typical day changed before and after Axiom pulled out of its acquisition attempt.

Organizational Roles

OB nurses at Fuller Hospital rotate weekly through several organizational positions in the unit: DR (delivery room—dated language since there are no designated "delivery rooms" in the unit), pairs (postpartum—mom and baby pairs), overflow unit (overflow postpartum unit), and charge nurse. The positions have priorities, too. For example, on a given day shift, there are typically three nurses assigned to labor patients: DR1, DR2, and DR3. The first labor patient, whether a woman who arrives at the hospital in spontaneous labor or scheduled for an induction, is assigned to the nurse who is DR1. The next labor patient is assigned to the nurse who is DR2, and so on. For a scheduled cesarean, a nurse who is unlikely to be assigned a labor patient in the next few hours (i.e., either a pairs nurse or the DR2 or DR3 nurse, depending on how many labor patients have been admitted) will scrub, circulate, or be assigned to the baby—the three roles nurses take for cesareans, although typically a NICU nurse is the baby nurse.[1] If a labor patient has an unscheduled cesarean, the DR nurse who was assigned to the patient will typically be the circulator and a pairs nurse will scrub in. The charge nurse or another nurse who has a light load will watch the pairs nurse's patients while the pairs nurse scrubs in for the cesarean.

The overflow unit—commonly referred to as 3 West—first opened in March 2015 to deal with the increased number of patients from the two new practices. It is not always open, and, thus, nurses may or may not be assigned to that unit. It is a good distance from the OB unit—about a seven-minute walk—and two nurses, at least one of whom is an RN, must always be assigned to the overflow unit if it is open.[2] Up to five postpartum patients and their babies can stay in the overflow unit. This is a case in which the LDRP routine is disrupted because women are moved to the overflow unit during their postpartum stay. Most patients do not like this move, and nurses use this to their advantage to encourage patients to leave the hospital early (i.e., be discharged) and free up an LDRP room for another patient. Tammy tells me, "[We tell patients], 'You might move your room twice,' and we're trying to be, like, 'Everything's great in here! Want to go home early?' We're, like, trying to . . . get people out sooner than they're supposed to because we don't have rooms for people."

Although the charge position is in the rotation, not all nurses are allowed to be in charge. To be charge nurse, the hospital requires the nurse to have been employed in the Fuller OB unit for a minimum of two years and to have completed specific training. Most nurses loathe being in charge. They are paid a small amount per hour in addition to their regular hourly wage, and that amount depends on the nurse's seniority. Most nurses told me that their extra pay is between $1.50 and $2.70 per hour. Nurses have a running joke that it is only a dollar per hour and they do not think the extra responsibilities and work are consummate with the additional pay. I overheard one nurse telling another nurse not to joke about the pay rate because if the nurse manager heard, she would get mad. The charge nurse is responsible for the entire unit. She assigns nurses to patients, makes sure all rooms are clean and stocked, and deals with staffing issues—putting nurses on call if there are too few patients, calling nurses on call to come in if there are too many patients, assigning patients to herself if there are no other available nurses, and ensuring that the next shift has adequate staffing. The charge nurse takes on a "pair" if needed. She is also the "default" nurse if on a given shift the nurse assigned to a certain slot in the rotation is not scheduled to work or calls out. The charge nurse is also responsible for updating the computers to reflect which nurse is assigned to which patients. She also coordinates care of patients and must communicate with physicians and midwives when there is no room for a patient, or with the physician or midwife and patient when, for example, a patient's induction must be rescheduled. The other job of a charge nurse is to ensure that new nurses are doing their jobs correctly, although from my observations it is rare for the charge nurse to directly supervise other nurses.

The charge position became more stressful over time as the hospital faced financial difficulties and patient loads increased. In one observation I conducted in January 2015, the charge nurse is assigned a postpartum patient who had hemorrhaged the night before. A hemorrhage patient requires intense care and oversight, and such a patient would typically not be assigned to the charge nurse. One nurse asks, "Why is Jennifer assigned to that room?" Another nurse answers, "There's no one else to take it." In other words, even patient safety came into question with organizational changes happening in the hospital.

Jamie told me about the stress of being charge nurse in our September 2015 interview:

Technically, it is all going to come back to me [as charge]. . . . I'm supposed to know everything that is going on. But as we've gotten way busier, it's a lot harder to do. . . . Some nights we work with everyone who has a lot of experience. So, we can multitask, and I don't have to think twice about it. And then there are nights where . . . three of the people I am working with have less than two years of experience. And it is very hard. And I don't expect them to know more. They should be allowed to do what they are doing, but the backup and support is really difficult when they don't have it.

Backup and support skills are essential in this unit where things can turn on a dime, and the charge nurse feels much stress when she cannot count on the nurses to have these skills.

One day in the breakroom over a snack, I asked Julie and Jennifer, two seasoned nurses, if they found it stressful to be charge nurse. Jennifer's emphatic answer: "Oh yeah." They continued in conversation, answering my questions along the way, and I share this exchange because it shows the level of frustration nurses feel being in charge. Note that part of their frustration is with demands by physicians who do not understand the constraints they face:

JULIE: It can be [stressful].
JENNIFER: *More* stressful.
JULIE: And, we get paid, what, a whole $1.50 an hour [more]?
JENNIFER: Yes. . . . It's not like you're not thinking of patients, too. You have [charge duties].
JULIE: Plus, you have a full patient assignment . . . if we're filling up.
JENNIFER: We're too busy to do all of that.
JULIE: If we're filling up and a c-section needs to be bumped, an induction needs to be bumped, you've got to call the doctors, coordinate this, call the patients. And nobody's ever happy with you.
JENNIFER: No. I tell you, you can tell them [physicians] you have no room. [They'll say,] "Well, this is ridiculous saying we have no room!"

JULIE: No room. You have to be pretty straightforward.

JENNIFER: And forget telling them you don't have the staff.

JULIE: Oh yeah. They don't even want to hear [that].

JENNIFER: Even concrete: We have no rooms. There's no bed to put a patient in.

It is clear that being in charge is stressful, and that the stress has only gone up.

My interview in November 2015 with Lori corroborates this analysis. She tells me, "Every time somebody comes in and says, 'You're charge,' . . . it's like, 'Oh fuck . . . I don't want to be in charge.' And . . . a lot of them [charge nurses] are, at the end of the shift, almost crying." I followed up by asking her if this was a change since the new practices started in March. She indicated that it was: "I mean we would have bad charge days, but . . . it wasn't a bad charge day *every day*."

Organizational Work Rules and Policies

OB nurses at Fuller work eight- or twelve-hour shifts, although more nurses work eight- rather than twelve-hour shifts and some nurses work a combination of eight- and twelve-hour shifts. The hospital has three eight-hour nursing shifts: day (7:00 a.m.–3:00 p.m.), evening (3:00 p.m.–11:00 p.m.), and night (11:00 p.m.–7:00 a.m.). Nurses who work twelve-hour shifts start at the beginning of a typical eight-hour shift, for example 7:00 a.m.–7:00 p.m., or at a time that allows them to end at a typical eight-hour shift, for example 11:00 a.m.–11:00 p.m. Full-time status requires a thirty-two-hour workweek and is desirable because the hospital pays a higher percentage of the nurse's health insurance premium if she is employed full-time and reimburses the nurse's educational expenses, for example if she seeks a graduate or professional degree or finishes a bachelor's degree (a number of the nurses do not have a four-year college degree). Nurses are employed for a specific shift (day, evening, or night), although they may cover a different shift if they sign up to cover for another nurse.

A common concern of nurses regarding the impending acquisition was that they would be forced to work twelve-hour shifts. For example, Jennifer tells me, "I've heard from other nurses that worked for a hospital that has merged, like, they're making everyone go to twelve-hour shifts." When I asked a unit administrator about this, she said it is likely that the new company would move all nurses to twelve-hour shifts if for no other reason that it is complicated to staff a unit with nurses who work different shift lengths—eight and twelve hours—because there are sometimes dangling, four-hour "princess shifts." She explained to me, "They're going to come in and look at things like that, and if they see the challenges that having all these crazy shifts creates, they might say, 'Enough of this. Let's just go to all twelves. . . . Those kinds of things come down from above and you just have to go with them." Another administrator told me that twelve-hour shifts are more efficient and allow more flexibility in scheduling. I asked her to explain how. She answered, "Well instead of having three shifts, you have two, so there's less overlapping time for report. There's more flexibility so that if somebody is working two twelve-hour shifts and getting their twenty-four hours in there . . . they could much more easily pick up another shift because there's so many other days in the week." However, the unit administrator who discussed the "princess shifts" expressed a concern that older nurses may not be able to physically meet the demands of a twelve-hour shift: "If they . . . tell me I've got to go back to the bedside, I'm going to be in trouble because, for older nurses, the twelve-hour shifts are really, probably, not safe even. For us to work beyond the eight-hour mark, we are now moving into a point of exhaustion, and we're not thinking clearly."

Given the efficiency and ease of scheduling twelve-hour shifts discussed above, it is not surprising that in the summer of 2015, *after* the Axiom acquisition fell through and while the hospital was trying to woo other potential hospital systems, the OB unit incentivized a twelve-hour-shift schedule. I see this as likely explained by administrators' desire to (1) experience the efficiency and flexibility indicated by the administrators above and (2) show potential suitors that they are making changes to become more efficient. The way unit administrators incentivized a twelve-hour shift was by introducing a cohort system. A cohort involves six nurses working twelve-hour shifts. Three of the nurses work a day shift (7 a.m.–7 p.m.) and three of the nurses work a night shift (7 p.m.–7 a.m.). The six nurses in the cohort work a combined total of 168 hours per week. Two nurses from each shift work thirty-two hours per week and one nurse from each shift works twenty hours per week. These per-week hours are averaged over three weeks. For example, the thirty-two-hour-shift nurses work two weeks of three twelve-hour shifts and one week of two twelve-hour shifts. This is a total of ninety-six hours over three weeks, which averages to thirty-two hours per week. Nurses who work a twenty-hour shift work two weeks of two twelve-hour shifts and one week of one twelve-hour shift. This totals sixty hours over three weeks, which averages to twenty hours per week. Cohorts have a three-week revolving schedule in which each nurse works every third weekend and, if they can find cooperative cohort members, nurses can arrange the schedule such that every three weeks, they have seven days off in a row. Initially, signing up to be in a cohort was based on seniority. However, cohort schedule availability proliferated over the next year so that even nurses with very little seniority could enter a cohort. Although it sounds and is, indeed, complicated, once the schedule is set, the three-week schedule rotates in a predictable way.

All registered nurses (RNs) are unionized, although licensed practical nurses (LPNs) and surgery techs are not, and many of the intricate rules that are laid out in the coming pages are a result of union rules. Nurses from other units in the hospital do not "float" into the OB unit to work when the unit is busy. The OB unit is considered closed in this way. Because the unit is closed and, thus, cannot draw nurses from other units when it gets busy, OB nurses are required to sign up to cover twelve hours of call each month in three four-hour shifts. This means they must sign up for an additional twelve hours each month for which they will be available to be called to work if the obstetric unit gets busy (referred to as required call or RC). The nurses are divided into three different groups—A, B, and C—and the order in which the groups are able to sign up for call rotates each month. Seniority is not factored into when a nurse signs up for call. The most unpopular required call shifts are 3:00 a.m.–7:00 a.m. and 11:00 p.m.–3:00 a.m. Many nurses sign up for call at the end of an assigned eight-hour shift so that, if they must take call, they just stay longer. Especially nurses who travel a significant distance to come to work use this strategy. Nurses are required to sign up for the same number of call hours, regardless of how many hours they are typically scheduled to work. Jennifer identified this as a problem: "The required call of a person who's scheduled sixteen hours part-time is the same amount as if you're working forty hours a week. . . . So, it [is] a lot. So, basically, you could end up working sixteen days in a row, if you got called in for your required calls. . . . It's not fun."

Besides having to sign up for required call, nurses may also be placed on call if the OB unit is not busy. The use of being "on call" to designate both nurses' being required to be available to work extra time and nurses' being required to leave a current shift was confusing to me, but these are two clear and distinct processes, and I rarely saw nurses get confused by what I would suggest is a fairly complicated system. However, the system apparently takes time to learn. When I expressed confusion over the system, one nurse told me, "I was here probably a good year before I really understood the mandatory call and the numbers in the call book." When a nurse is required to leave a current shift because the OB unit is not busy, she writes down the date and the number of hours she lost in the call book, which is kept at the front desk. This record is kept for all nurses and resets on January 1 of each year.[3] When the charge nurse decides that all scheduled nurses are not needed, she first asks if anyone wants to leave and be put on call (requested call). If no one volunteers, she goes to the call book and sees, of the nurses working, who has the fewest hours of call since the beginning of the year and places that nurse on call. If two nurses on the shift have the same number of hours for which they have been placed on call, the charge nurse will put on call the nurse whose last call was on the earlier date. Being placed on call means that the nurse must clock out but must be available to be called back in if the OB unit gets busy. This means she must be ready to work (e.g., she may not consume alcohol or go too far from the hospital).

Although the OB unit does not accept "floater" nurses from other units, nurses from the OB unit may float to another unit rather than being placed on call. If a nurse is told she is being placed on call for her shift and the nurse offers to float but there are no positions in the hospital for her to "float to," she will be mandated to take call, referred to as mandatory call or MC. That means she does not have a choice and will be placed on call. A nurse may not be asked to take mandatory call more than three times in one quarter. Mandatory call works differently for holidays. A nurse who has been mandated to take call on one holiday may not be mandated to take call on another holiday if there is another nurse working who has not taken mandatory call on a holiday in the current calendar year. These rules have been developed to promote fairness in terms of the number of hours worked and pay lost due to a nurse's taking mandatory call. Nurses are paid at a higher rate for holidays, hence the rules that focus specifically on holidays.

However, regardless of how intricate the rules are and how they cover almost every foreseeable circumstance, it was also clear to me that rules are sometimes made on the fly. In one instance, the charge nurse posted on the nurses' closed Facebook page the need for nurses to come in and help, which a secretary pointed out to her was in violation of the rules. Another time, a nurse was frustrated because she was required the day before to take mandatory call, but she had already been put on mandatory call the maximum number of times allowed in the quarter. She asked to float, but the charge nurse told her that another nurse being put on call had called back first and had taken the only float position available. The nurse asked, "Is this a new rule? The problem is that nurses sometimes are making these rules up as they go." The established rule allows a nurse who had been put on call the maximum times allowed in the quarter to be given the opportunity to float before any other nurses are allowed to float.

The on-call arrangement benefits the hospital by allowing flexible staffing; however, the arrangement does not guarantee nurses a minimum number of hours per week and, further, leads to unpredictable work hours. For example, nurses on call receive only seven dollars per hour, more than two dollars below the state's minimum hourly wage. Nurses are often critical of this situation. In discussing the unit, Julie brings up her frustration with being placed on call. She tells me:

> We are possessive of our time, and nobody wants to stay on call. We just want to work our hours. And it's basically the hospital and the higher-ups going, "You know what, if you're overstaffed, someone needs to stay home." Why can't people just work their hours? . . . Honesty, there's plenty on this unit [to do].

Julie goes on to tell me that because the unit does not have nursing assistants—all the nurses are RNs or LPNs—their unit has more "call offs." She tells me that this "comes down to money." RNs and LPNs cost more than aides. She continues, "If we had less nurses and more aides, we wouldn't get called off [as much]."

It is ultimately the charge nurse's decision about whether and how many nurses should be put on call. I asked several nurses what happens if the charge nurse does not put enough nurses on call. I was told that the nurse manager would "talk to" the charge nurse. One nurse told me that the nurse manager had called her once and told her that she was wasting money by keeping so many nurses on when the patient load was low. The dilemma for charge nurses is that they have the responsibility of staffing the unit in the face of patient loads that can change quickly. Thus, they experience both pressure not to overstaff but the worry, too, of understaffing and the potential drastic consequences of not having enough nurses in the unit. Debbie, a nurse with many years of experience, explains:

> In OB, you never know from one minute to the next what's going to happen. Three people can walk in, in labor in five minutes. . . . You . . . can't staff for "what if." But you have to have enough [nurses] that it's safe. . . . Sometimes there's empty spots on the schedule, and no one's willing to come in. On the other hand, you can get pressure from management to go down and not have so many people. You have to think about it. You have to negotiate with your staff, and you have to be flexible. Sometimes it can be okay, but, sometimes, not being at the top is, it's a hard world.

Another nurse told me that even if you aren't "talked to" about keeping nurses on unnecessarily and wasting money, there is a more general worry that the hospital administration will fire or lay off nurses. In other words, the "talking to" doesn't need to happen for nurses to worry.

If a nurse who is scheduled to work is put on call and then called back to work, she is paid seven dollars per hour on top of her normal hourly wage. In this way nurses are compensated for the disruption to their schedule, and their scheduled hours are somewhat protected. Yet the charge nurse bears the responsibility of having increased the cost of labor for the unit. Julie tells me that management also talks to charge nurses for having to call back nurses who were put on mandatory call:

> You do hear it from the managers. . . . The problem is when you put someone on call, they go on call, which is seven dollars an hour. And, if they get called back in, they'll continue to get their extra seven dollars an

hour now on top of their regular pay. So, they're actually more expensive sometimes putting them on call and getting called back. It's a gamble.

I noted that the call schedule also may negatively affect nurses who take another nurse's shift or switch shifts with another nurse. One nurse was very angry one day because she was put on call during a shift she was working for another nurse (they had switched shifts). She said, "I can't believe I switched and ended up being put on call!"

Another policy worth discussion relates to vacation. Time off during "prime vacation time," defined as the beginning of June through the middle of September, is contentious. The vacation sign-up is listed by shift—day, evening, and night. The signup is arranged by seniority in terms of hospital (not unit) employment, with the most senior nurses listed at the top of the sheet and the most junior nurse at the bottom. Only two nurses on a given shift are allowed to take vacation on the same day, and nurses may take only two weeks of vacation during prime time, even if they have more vacation weeks owed to them, which is not unusual. Nurses sometimes cooperate directly or indirectly. One nurse mentioned that her birthday is the same week as the birthday of another nurse's daughter. She tries to avoid taking the week of her birthday for vacation so that the other nurse can have time to celebrate with her young daughter.

I also convey in this section the many duties of a nurse and the complexity of the job. I was often asked during my observations if I was conducting my research because I had a secret desire to be a nurse. My standard answer: "No way! This job is too hard!" I am quite certain my description of what nurses do daily will make it clear to the reader why I answered this way.

Nurses tend to arrive ten or fifteen minutes before their shift starts. The closest parking lot is available to employees, patients, and visitors. This is sometimes problematic for nurses because the lot becomes full. Nurses, then, must park much farther away. Such a situation arose during one of my observations. An OB unit secretary complained that she had to wait five minutes to get a parking spot and, even then, had to park a "long ways away." She told everyone at the desk, "I'll have to have my keys out for protection when I walk to my car this evening." When my observations ended after dark, it was typical for the nurse I shadowed to ask where I parked and, if we were in the same lot, to suggest we walk together. In other words, worrying about walking to the parking lot at night, especially if one's car was in the back of the lot, was common. As I mentioned above, the OB unit is located on the third floor of the building. Most nurses take the stairs, but there is an elevator. The OB unit is locked. Hospital employees and volunteers must scan their IDs to open and unlock the door. Visitors must pick up a telephone receiver on the wall and ask to be let in. This receiver rings at the front desk, and either a secretary or nurse answers by asking, "Who are you here to see?"

Until a policy change in June 2016, nurses in the unit could wear scrubs they purchased for themselves or hospital-furnished scrubs in a light blue or deep plum color. In 2015, the OB unit administrators instituted a new policy that nurses must wear hospital-furnished scrubs in the OR. A unit administrator told me that this change was prompted by a new guideline from the Association of periOperative Registered Nurses (AORN). Before this rule was implemented, nurses were allowed to wear their owns scrubs and to wear a sterile white jumpsuit over their scrubs if they went into the OR. During the period before this change, most nurses chose to buy their own scrubs and to wear a sterile jumpsuit or change into the hospital scrubs if they went into the OR. Nurses who bought their own scrubs had a choice in their style and color or pattern. Nurses would often remark on the scrubs of other nurses with comments like "That color is so cute!" and "Where did you find that top?" and "I love that shade of turquoise!" Some nurses also spent time during the day shopping for scrubs online, sometimes during break and sometimes not. At times, I observed nurses as a group spending fifteen minutes or more behind the front desk engrossed in looking at online scrub sites. In general, I found that because most nurses picked their own scrubs, there was a focus on how fashionable the scrubs were.

In June 2016 the policy changed again, and nurses in the unit are now required to wear hospital-laundered scrubs *at all times*. They have a choice of light blue or plum scrubs, although some nurses wear green scrubs from the OR. This change in policy was prompted by an unresolved postoperative infection spike in which eleven women contracted post-cesarean infections over a short time period. Implementing this scrub policy is one of the ways unit administrators were addressing the infection outbreak. Cynthia, one of the administrators, told me that the policy change was long overdue and that at other hospitals nurses must wear hospital-laundered scrubs. She told me that having nurses wear hospital-laundered scrubs in the OR was part of an effort to reduce the infection rate, but that it was also costing the hospital money:

> We're talking about having to buy . . . all new scrubs because we're chang-ing the process for the way people dress when they go into the OR in order to see if that's part of the [infection] problem. So, we're spending money on that for this infection rate issue and . . . someone in a manage-ment position, who has a budget that they have to deal with, they're going to . . . feel the extra pressure. You know . . . I'm going to have to take from Peter to pay Paul, and . . . what does that do to Peter? . . . That is more stressful at a time like this, without a doubt.

Yet the policy change was likely warranted. I have observational notes for January 2014 in which one of the nurses put on a sterile white jump-suit to cover her scrubs in preparation to help with a cesarean. The surgery was delayed and she came to the front desk and chatted with the other nurses. During the conversation, she dropped her mask on the floor, picked it up, and reused it. In other words, the white suit and mask were certainty not sterile when she returned to the operating room.

A nurse locker room is located outside the unit but on the same floor. During my observational period, most nurses did not use it, instead storing coats and personal items in the break room. However, in the last few months of my observations, the nurse manager made a new rule that coats must be left in the locker room. When nurses arrive on the unit, they used to head to the break room, but now most nurses stop in the locker room to put their coats away. Yet, after this new rule was established, some nurses continued to place their coats on the counter in the break room. Nurses then often grab a cup of coffee in the break room. The physicians affiliated with the OB unit of Fuller Hospital give a subscription for "good" coffee as a holiday gift to the nurses. The cof-fee is delivered regularly in large boxes to the break room. When the good coffee runs out between orders, it is a common topic of discussion among the nurses, who speak of being out of good coffee with derision and frustration. Several of the nurses mentioned the good coffee sub-scription to me as a perk.

There is also a seldom-used Keurig coffee maker and a toaster on the counter in the break room. I witnessed an interesting interaction during one of my later observation periods. A rather taciturn physician from one of the new practices came in the break room and used the Keurig to make a cup of coffee. A doctor from one of the established offices told him that the coffee in the pot isn't that bad. The new doctor said, in a rather chilly tone, "I find that taste is mostly affected by one's company." This shows a passive-aggressive stance between the two practices and is an anecdotal example of how the pinches of organizational change affected a wide variety of actors in the hospital.

After the nurse gets whatever coffee, tea, or other beverage she plans to drink for her shift (many nurses keep in the break room cups that are labeled with their names), she clocks in electronically on a device located on the wall in the hallway just around the corner from the door to the break room. She then heads to the front desk. There is a dry-erase board on the wall just outside the break room and above where the nurses clock in that indicates who is the charge nurse (i.e., who is "in charge") on each shift. This information is also kept on a clipboard at the front desk. In fact, the clipboard is the master plan, so to speak, with room numbers and nurse assignments. The electronic chart is updated when the charge nurse or another nurse helping out changes it. If the floor is busy, the electronic chart may not be updated for some time.

If the nurse is assigned a patient when she begins her shift, she "receives report" from the nurse who took care of the patient on the previous shift. During most of my observational period, nurses sometimes gave report to the incoming nurse in the patient's room, but more often nurses gave report at the front or back desk or sometimes in the break room. Toward the end of my observational period, the nurse manager instituted a rule that nurses may not give report in a public space, including at the front and back desks. This rule was designed both to protect patient health information and to cut down on noise at the front desk. However, the rule was not always followed. In the process of "giving report," the nurses look together over the chart, including the prenatal record, and the outgoing nurse presents any pertinent information about the chart or about the medical care the patient has received. If the patient is in labor, the presenting nurse goes over basic information about the patient's age, marital status, number of pregnancies (gravidity) and births (parity), and the status of labor (e.g., Has there been a vaginal exam to check cervical dilation, and, if so, when? Are the membranes intact or ruptured? If they are ruptured, is the amniotic fluid clear or were there signs of meconium—the baby's first poop, which, if done in utero, can be aspirated by the baby at birth?). She communicates about when the last vital signs were taken and, if Pitocin is being given, when it was last increased and what the current level is. If the woman has an epidural, the nurse indicates when the epidural was placed and how it is working. The outgoing nurse also summarizes the fetal heartbeat and contraction patterns. Typically, the outgoing nurse also mentions whether anyone is or has been in the room with the patient (e.g., husband, partner, friend, parent). If the patient is postpartum, the outgoing nurse goes over details of the birth (when it occurred, whether it was vaginal or a cesarean, and any complications); the sex and name of the baby; when she last took vital signs of the woman and baby; when discharge is likely to happen; if discharge papers have been completed; whether, if necessary, paternity papers have been completed; if there are any remaining newborn assessments to be completed; and, if the baby is a boy, if a circumcision has been done or, if not, if the parents would like the baby to be circumcised.

If a new laboring patient is assigned to the nurse, she first looks for the patient's prenatal record. I observed nurses spending quite a bit of time looking for prenatal records and, if they could not find one for a patient, asking the secretary to call the patient's OB practice to have it faxed over. Sometimes the secretary is busy or not at the desk, and the nurse calls the practice herself. One of the group practices installed software at the front desk on the "doctor/midwife computer," which gave the group's physicians and midwives electronic access to the prenatal records, but only one group practice had this ability and the nurses still could not access the prenatal records without the help of a midwife or physician from the group. Once the nurse has the prenatal record, she reads it carefully to see how it will affect the patient's care. For example, if the patient is group-B strep (GBS) positive, the patient will receive a course of antibiotics to prevent the infection from spreading to the baby, which could cause a life-threating condition. If the patient has a history of postpartum depression, drug dependence, or a mental-health issue, the nurse will set up a visit from a social worker before the patient is discharged. She also looks for marital status. If the patient is not married, the nurse discusses paternity with the patient, because if the father is known and present he will be asked to sign paternity papers (to submit to the state) before the baby is discharged. The nurse also checks to make sure test results for rubella, hepatitis B, and HIV have been recorded in the prenatal record and that two blood screens for blood type have been completed (done in case of a blood transfusion).

Once the patient is admitted to the unit, the nurse can put into the computer a plan of care for either a vaginal or a cesarean birth. However, she needs to speak to a physician or midwife to ask him/her to put in *orders* to take care of the patient. If the conversation takes place over the phone, the physician or midwife authorizes the nurse to put in orders in the name of the physician or midwife. These orders authorize, for example, fetal heart monitoring, contraction monitoring, and taking the patient's vital signs.

If the nurse is assigned a new labor patient who has not yet been admitted, she collects or verifies information from the patient about insurance status, address, medical history, health information (allergies, vaccinations, vitamins, medications, whether she has been exposed to TB or Ebola, and, oddly enough, whether the patient is pregnant), history of alcohol and drug consumption, history of smoking, and information about anxiety and postpartum depression, whether the patient had prenatal education, and what pediatrician the patient has chosen for the baby. She asks the patient if she has been exposed to anything contagious, whether she has a plan for labor, if she plans to breast- or bottle-feed, and, if the baby is known to be a boy, if she wants to have the baby circumcised. She also asks about her religious preference and if she has any beliefs that affect her care. She ends with questions about family support, newborn experience, and living arrangements.

Nurses receive help with many of these tasks from the secretaries (the term used in the hospital for this position). During most of my observational period, two secretaries worked on the day shift , and one secretary worked on the evening shift. The night-shift nurses, because the floor was quieter—no scheduled cesareans and few inductions to start—are believed to have time to deal with secretarial issues, although that is not always the case because some nights are quite busy. Secretaries also rotated weekends so that a secretary is on duty during the day on weekends. This all changed significantly in November 2015 when secretarial hours were cut across the hospital. Suddenly nurses on all shifts were overwhelmed with what would typically have been secretarial tasks—admitting patients, finding prenatal records, calling the lab to ask someone to come to the unit to pick up blood that has been drawn, calling engineering about broken equipment, and so forth.[4]

After the nurse receives report and/or reviews the prenatal record and the physician or midwife submits an order for the patient, the nurse can care for the patient. She takes the patient's temperature and blood pressure (i.e., vital signs). The blood pressure is automatically documented on the patient's electronic record, but the temperature is not. The nurse may document in the room—there is a small laptop computer in each room on a built-in shelf and desk area that is to the left or right of the head of the patient's bed—or she may write the information down and chart at a computer at the main or back desk. Before leaving the room, nurses almost always ask patients if they need anything and remind patients to push the call button if they need something when the nurse is not in the room.

If the patient has an epidural, the nurse may suggest to the patient that she sleep until her labor is further along. If the patient follows this suggestion, the nurse may turn out the lights and perhaps draw the shades. The nurse then watches the electronic fetal monitoring strip from the front desk, where nurses are able to pull up the live monitoring strips of the patients on a computer. However, whether the patient is sleeping or awake, the nurse regularly goes to the room to check on the patient and to document the patient's vital signs and, depending on the patient, to check the patient's IV fluids, monitor the epidural, turn up the Pitocin, and/or administer fluids, antibiotics, or other medication.

If the physician or midwife decides to administer a cervical ripener vaginally (to begin an induction), the nurse fills the order and accompanies the physician or midwife when the cervical ripener is inserted into the patient's vagina. Similarly, the nurse also almost always accompanies the physician or midwife when it is decided to break the patient's water or check cervical dilation. Sometimes the nurse checks the patient's dilation, but it is more typical for the physician or midwife to do this.

Physicians and midwives order Pitocin for some patients. Pitocin is an artificial form of oxytocin, the chemical a woman's body produces that causes uterine contractions. If the physician or midwife decides to administer Pitocin, he or she will ask the nurse to fill the order and administer it. This is also the case with almost any type of medication. Nurses are responsible for administering most drugs. Pitocin may be given to induce labor, to augment contractions, or both. If a woman is given Pitocin, she will be monitored more carefully because Pitocin can cause tachysystole (i.e., hyper stimulation of the uterus), which can lead to fetal distress. In fact, I observed such a situation unfold during one of my observations. The patient was fully dilated and pushing, but the doctor was impatient (and had been throughout the patient's labor). The nurse, trying to facilitate a vaginal birth for the patient and having to go to extra lengths because of the doctor's hurry, offers to start Pitocin (often referred to as "Pit") to increase the frequency of the patient's contractions in hopes of getting her to deliver more quickly. However, when the nurse starts Pitocin, the fetal heart rate decreases to dangerously low levels.[5] What follows is an excerpt from my field notes:

> Kim [the nurse] asks the physician, "Do you want me to grab some Pit? I have some." The physician says to the patient, "We're going to add medication to give strength to your contractions." Kim comes back with tubes [for the Pitocin]. The physician says, "You seem to be pushing fine." Kim tells the patient they need the contractions to come more quickly because the baby's head goes back up between the contractions. . . . Kim asks [the patient] if she wants water or ice cubes. The patient says she's okay for now. . . . Kim [starts Pitocin and] documents this on the computer in the room. The baby's heart rate drops into the sixties. Panic ensues! The physician says she [the patient] needs an internal monitor. Kim takes out the oxygen mask, puts it on the patient, and they role her to her side. Kim pushes an alarm button next to the patient's bed, and three more nurses and a pediatrician rush into the room. The pediatrician prepares the crib. They struggle to get the internal monitor to work. They switch cords, and finally it works. Sandra [one of the nurses who came running in] announces the fetal heart rate: sixties, eighties, sixties, nineties . . . They turn off the Pit. The baby starts to sound better [the fetal heart rate increases]. Kim tells the patient that the baby is being squeezed and doesn't like that. . . . The physician suggests that the patient push on her side. . . . Kim says, "So much for Pit. The Pit was on for thirteen seconds."

The situation documented in my field notes is an example of why women given Pitocin are carefully monitored. This vigilance entails a special focus on the electronic fetal monitor (to make sure the fetus is tolerating the Pitocin), and the toco (tocodynamometer), which measures the duration and presence of contractions, to ensure the contractions are not lasting too long or coming too frequently.

The nurse's responsibility for filling a medication order involves several steps. First, the physician or midwife puts the order into the computer, and the pharmacy approves the order electronically. Often nurses have to remind physicians and midwives to put in a medication order. Second, the nurse goes to the medication room, a small, secure stockroom. She logs into the computer that sits atop a metal cabinet with several small drawers and searches for the patient's record. If everything works right, which is not always the case, the medication will be linked to the patient's ID. When she requests the ordered and approved medication (on the computer screen), one of the small drawers in the cabinet under the computer pops open (literally—it can be quite startling if one is not expecting it!), and the nurse takes the medication out of the drawer.[6] She then takes the medication to the room.

Once the nurse brings the medication to the patient's room, she must scan her ID, the patient's identification bracelet, and the medication before she can administer the medication to the patient. Scanning is a patient-safety check to make sure the right patient is being given the right medication (called bedside medication verification), but the scans can fail, and this failure causes nurses much frustration, something I saw countless times. Another frustration I saw was in nurses' forgetting to scan the medication until they had already taken it out of its individual packaging thus destroying the code that needs to be scanned. This required the nurse to fetch the packaging from the trash, straighten it out, and override the system. If this failed, she had to go back to the stockroom to get more medication. In fact, in my observations it was rare for this patient-safety practice to go without a glitch, and this covers the time from implementation in the summer of 2013 through my final observations in June 2016. In May 2014, a day I followed Julie, an IT staff member was trying to fix the scanning system in one of the rooms. Julie tells me, "Every time they introduce something new, it causes problems." When I asked her what problems she specifically saw in the medication scanning system, she tells me, "It doesn't scan or it freezes. Everything they do causes a problem." In January 2015 Lillian tells me, after not being able to scan her patient's Pitocin bag, "It's really a patient-safety issue to make sure the right patient has the right medicine. It's a last-minute safety check. But it's not very helpful if it doesn't scan." Evelyn tries to joke with a patient when the scanner doesn't work, saying "I'm doing groceries here, right?" She has to override the system twice when the bar code of the medication she is giving the patient is not found in the system. Further, the scanners sometimes go missing. In a May 2014 observation, the secretary asked nurses to check every room to see which was missing a scanner, because a scanner had shown up at the front desk. It is important to note that this new protocol increases the nurses' work in other ways as well. If the system were implemented in such a way that the medication, when scanned, automatically read into the patient's electronic record, that could at least be seen as making the nurse's tasks easier. But it does not. Sylvia tells me, "Even though we scan the patient and we scan the medication, I still have to put it in the chart . . . It's just not part of the system."

Nurses give most patients IV fluids. This is always the case if the patient has an epidural because epidurals often cause a woman's blood pressure to drop. Increased fluids mediate this effect. Yet most women without epidurals are also given IV fluids. In fact, it was rare in my observations for a woman in labor not to have an IV for fluids. The fluid bag needs to be changed when it is empty. When the bag is empty, the pump beeps (this beeping also happens when epidural medication or Pitocin runs out or when the pump detects an air bubble in the line). Beeping "machines" are a common reason nurses are called to a patient's room, although sometimes patients try to solve the problem themselves by turning the beeping machine off. This frustrates nurses, who typically tell patients not to do that again since the nurses need to know the reason for the beeping. Nurses also spend a great deal of time untangling cords and tubes. This may sound silly to mention, but I observed it so often. There are cords from the electronic fetal monitor and toco as well as tubes for Pitocin, fluid, and/or medication. The cords and tubes need to be untangled if the patient gets up to walk or to use the bathroom. Patients who have an epidural do not have this problem because they are not allowed out of the bed once the epidural is administered.

A nurse assigned to a labor patient may do various things to facilitate the dilation of the patient's cervix and/or to increase the patient's comfort. For example, she may help the patient change positions, or she may offer to help her use a birth ball (a yoga-type ball on which a woman sits during labor) or peanut ball (an inflatable that looks like a peanut, which can be placed between a woman's legs while she lies on her side to help open her pelvic cavity during labor). The nurse may offer ice cubes or popsicles, get the woman socks, or help her to the bathroom. She often changes the pad underneath the patient when the patient is out of bed to make sure she always has a clean bed. The nurse may also encourage the patient to walk, especially in early labor, and may hook up a telemetry unit, which allows the nurse, doctor, and/or midwife to monitor the fetal heart rate and the patient's contraction pattern remotely. The nurse continues to take vital signs and attend to the patient as she labors. This includes keeping the physician or midwife responsible for the patient up to date.

All of this information is documented; in fact, nurses spend an inordinate amount of time on paperwork. Sylvia, an experienced nurse who had spent years documenting on paper before electronic records took hold, told one of her patients, "We're the paperwork Nazis!" The nurse must document every procedure the patient undergoes as well as the patient's and the fetus's condition. The primary focus in terms of monitoring the fetus is on the fetal heart rate. Most patients have continuous fetal heart monitoring, but some nurses will encourage the use of, or patients will ask for, intermittent monitoring, where the fetal heart rate is checked at defined times, typically every thirty minutes during the first stage of labor (cervical dilation) and every fifteen minutes during the second stage of labor (pushing). The nurse also monitors the patient's vital signs—temperature and blood pressure—and contraction pattern. If the patient has not ruptured her amniotic sac, a nurse will take the patient's temperature every four hours; if it is ruptured, a nurse will take her temperature every two hours. How often blood pressure is taken depends on whether the patient has an epidural, something that can lead to a rapid drop in blood pressure. If the patient has an epidural or certain health condition, the nurse will set the machine to automatically take the patient's blood pressure every fifteen minutes. If the patient does not have an epidural, the nurse will set the blood pressure to be checked every two to four hours in early labor, depending on whether the patient has any underlying issues, and every thirty minutes in active labor.

The nurse further documents any medical procedure, such as the patient's receiving an epidural or being induced, as well as any medication, such as epidural medication, Pitocin, or even Tylenol or Motrin. If the patient has an IV and is being administered fluid or an antibiotic, nurses document this and sometimes the patient's intake/output fluid chart. Nurses also make notes on the patient's chart about such things as the patient's pain level (on a scale of one to ten), whether the patient seems comfortable, and who is in the room with the patient. Nurses are able to "mark" the electronic strip that displays a timeline of the fetal heart rate and the patient's contraction record by pushing a button on the monitor. Marking puts a vertical line on the patient's "strip" (both the physical and electronic strip) at the exact time the nurse presses the "mark" button. This enables her to go back and make an electronic notation on the patient's record. The marking feature is especially useful if the nurse is too busy to document on the electronic strip in real time.

Sometime during the patient's labor, the nurse makes sure the crib warmer works and gets the crib ready for delivery—laying blankets out and making sure the oxygen is working. She also makes sure the baby thermometer is present and working. She finds a baby scale and places it just outside the room or in the room. Some hospitals have an integrated crib and scale. Although this hospital does have integrated cribs and scales in the ORs and in the NICU, the LDRP rooms do not have these—the cribs and scales are separate. If there is not a spotlight in the room, the nurse will look around the unit to find one. The spotlight is used at the time of birth for the physician or midwife to have ample light to see the baby as it is born. The nurse also sets up the delivery table, which has a cabinet below that houses two shelves. As part of setting it up, she counts the pairs of scissors, the sponges, and the clamps, which are all placed on top of the table. Unit administrators instituted a new rule in 2015 that nurses must obtain the signature of another nurse that the sponges have been counted correctly. Nurses loathe this rule and routinely skirt it by simply securing another nurse's signature without having her actually count the sponges. Rumor has it that this new rule is due to a particular physician twice leaving sponges inside a patient, something they say has nothing to do with their count but is due to the physician's carelessness. One nurse who talked to me about the new policy said, "My frustration is that they aren't holding the doctor accountable at all. The doctor probably didn't hear about it or barely heard about it. It just increased *my* work." After the nurse sets up the delivery table, she covers it with a sterile sheet.

The goal of labor is for the patient's cervix to dilate to a diameter of ten centimeters. Until that goal is reached, which can be hours or even days, nurses continue to take care of the patient by monitoring the fetal heart rate and the woman's contraction pattern, by taking and recording vital signs and the status of the woman and fetus, by changing the bags of fluid, Pitocin, epidural medication, and/or other medication, by documenting everything, by attending to the medical needs of the patient, and by trying to facilitate cervical dilation. I should note, too, that at any time a cesarean may be performed for any number of reasons, such as fetal distress, stalled labor (sometimes called failure to progress), or a woman's medical issues.

Once the cervix reaches ten centimeters' dilation, the patient starts to push the baby out. If a patient has an epidural, some, but not all, nurses encourage passive descent or "laboring down," which means the patient continues to labor without pushing until she feels pressure and/or the urge to push. Or the patient may be given a specified amount of time to labor down. To accomplish laboring down, the nurse may turn down or off the epidural and wait for the patient to have more feeling in her pelvis before she starts pushing. Some nurses swear by this practice and how it makes vaginal delivery more likely, especially for patients who have an epidural. When the patient feels pressure, the urge to push, or reaches the allotted time, the doctor or midwife reexamines the patient to see if the fetal head has descended to a lower position in the woman's pelvis.

Ideally, the nurse stays with the patient for almost the entire time the patient is pushing, which can be just a few minutes or can stretch to three or four hours. Nurses frequently eat a snack or meal just before a woman is fully dilated because it may be several hours before they have a break. The nurse is very busy during this phase of labor. She continues to monitor the patient's vital signs and contractions as well as the fetal heart rate. She also continues to chart. She is often the patient's cheerleader and almost always the director, by which I mean she talks the patient through pushing, telling her when to push (necessary if the patient's epidural keeps her from feeling her contractions), how long to push, and how to push. Sometimes she may put her fingers just touching the patient's perineum and ask the patient to push her fingers out. Or she may suggest that the patient push like she is having a bowel movement.

When birth becomes imminent, the nurse helps the physician or midwife put on sterile gloves and a sterile gown. The midwife or physician puts on the sterile gown over his or her scrubs, and the nurse secures the two sets of ties behind the robe to hold it on. The nurse also "breaks down" the bed. This involves removing the lower third of the bed to make it easier for the physician or midwife to help the women deliver her baby. She stores this removed part of the bed so it is out of the way, usually leaning it against a wall. When delivery is imminent, the nurse calls for a second nurse to provide care for the baby upon delivery. After the baby is born, the nurse calls the secretary to tell her the time of delivery. Soon after, the secretary brings to the patient's room bracelets for the baby (which also has an embedded security chip), the mother, and a significant other, which have the baby's identification number on them.

After the birth, the nurse cleans everything up and puts it in order, while still monitoring the woman and newborn. This is a clear distinction between doctors and nurses. Doctors leave as soon as sutures for any tears or an episiotomy are performed and the patient is stable. Nurses stay and take care of everything else for the baby, the mom, and the room. The nurse makes sure the baby is stable and healthy, she cleans the mother with wash clothes and, if the patient would like, she helps the patient into a clean gown. She reattaches the lower third of the bed that was removed for the birth. She helps the mother to hold the baby and, if she is breastfeeding, to latch the baby. After a bit of time, anywhere from thirty minutes or so to a few hours, the nurse will wash the baby for the first time.

However, her focus cannot just be on the patient and newborn. She also has a room to get in order. She accounts for all the instruments and sponges on the delivery table. She secures the placenta in a red bag and places it in a "placenta container" on the bottom of the delivery table. She places all dirty linens in a receptacle (a.k.a. laundry hamper) and makes sure the floor is reasonably clean, with no visible signs of blood. If it is not, she wipes up the floor as best as she can without a mop. After the pair is settled and doing well, the nurse carries the soiled linen receptacle and often a trash bag out of the room and down the back hall to the trash/waste room. These are quite heavy, and it is not unusual to see a nurse dragging two large bags behind her down the hall.

The nurse also drops the placenta container at the front desk to be picked up by a volunteer, who will take it to the lab. I should mention that it was not uncommon for these placentas to accumulate at the front desk. They sit on the top of the desk near the secretary, visible to all who walk by, although most people probably do not realize that placentas are in the bags. I often observed red bags at the desk. In fact, one day in January 2014 a day-shift secretary arrived at the hospital at 7:30 a.m. to find three placenta bags that had been at the desk since 3:00 p.m. the day before. She was angry and said that the evening-shift secretary should have taken them to the lab. A nurse defends the secretary, saying she was probably busy and it was just a "slip." The secretary arranges for them to be picked up. I am astounded that placentas—organs that have only recently been detached from women's bodies—have been sitting on a desk in the unit for more than twelve hours!

After the patient and room are clean, the nurse cleans the monitor and its cords and removes them from the room. They are on wheels, and she will either move them into a supply closet (located throughout the unit) or, if there is no room in a supply closet, to the end of the back hall in front of the window. The room now looks less like a labor room and more like a postpartum room.

One last task the nurse does is go to a cabinet in the nursery and retrieve a decorated card on which she writes the baby's first name, weight, and birth date. Nurses decorate these cards during slow times. She fills this card out and places it in the baby's crib. She continues to monitor the woman and baby until her shift ends. This includes doing the baby's "eyes and thighs" (vitamin K ointment for the eyes and a hepatitis B shot—standard treatment for babies unless the parents specifically opt out) and making its footprints in ink. Depending on her assignment, she may also be assigned to one or more other baby and mother pairs, a new labor patient, or a triage patient.

When the patient is ready to get out of bed, sometimes as long as twelve hours after the birth if the woman had an epidural or sooner if the patient is unmedicated, the nurse finds another nurse to come with her to get the patient to her feet. The nurse assigned to the patient helps the patient to the restroom, usually holding a quilted bed pad between her legs to prevent blood from dripping onto the floor. She helps the patient rinse her perineum and check for blood clots and instructs her to watch for blood clots that are "bigger than a plum." She then helps her into mesh underwear, a sanitary pad, and a fresh gown. While she is doing all of this, the second nurse fixes the bed. She strips the sheet, retrieves a padded plastic mattress from the closet, and puts that on top of the bed's mattress. She then makes the bed with fresh sheets in time for the patient to lie down when she returns from the bathroom.

It may seem that nurses assigned to a pair (i.e., a mom and baby) postpartum have an easy job, but I would suggest that this is not the case. They have several newborn screens they must complete, and some of the screens, especially the hearing screen, are onerous to complete. These screens include tests for hearing, cystic fibrosis, and congenital heart defects as well as a bilirubin screen. The woman and baby must also be regularly assessed and, if the woman is breastfeeding, the nurse must make sure the baby is feeding adequately.[7] The hospital uses a LATCH (latch, audible swallowing, type of nipple, comfort, hold/positioning) score to assess breastfeeding. Each assessment in the LATCH metric is given a score of zero, one, or two, and the scores are summed. The goal is to get a LATCH score of seven or better. If the woman and baby attain a score of at least seven three times in a row, the nurse can stop evaluating the baby's breastfeeding. The nurse also arranges for and assists the physician in circumcising (referred to as "circing") the baby if the baby is a boy and the parents want that done.

Nurses also deal with a great deal of paperwork involving the baby. This is not just documenting the care of the baby and the various screenings. The nurse must also deal with the baby's health insurance and give the parents paperwork to complete for the baby's social security number and birth certificate. If the parents are not married, an extra responsibility given to nurses is to discuss with the patient having the father of the baby sign paternity papers. When the father of the baby is present, they typically sign the papers and have the secretary notarize them. Nurses take this job seriously. One nurse told me that it is the state's way of making sure that dads pay for their kids. She saw this as important and fair and made sure to note the importance of paternity papers to patients.

There are also numerous other tasks that must be done for the unit, and all nurses are expected to help. For example, there is a "blue sheet" that has a list of things that must be checked off at the beginning of every shift (e.g., Is the OR stocked and ready to go? Are the glucose monitors clean?). "Doing the blue sheet" is not assigned to any one particular nurse but is to be completed by nurses who have time to do it. Restocking is also a never-ending process in the unit that must be done. Furthermore, disposing of outdated medications and supplies must be done periodically. These are all things nurses are expected to do when they "have time." Trips to the lab are also sometimes necessary. Although volunteers are typically available to take blood samples to the lab, sometimes nurses must go to the lab themselves. For example, I followed Sylvia to the lab one day to get a RhoGAM shot for a patient.[8] Nurses are assigned to give these shots or to evaluate a triage patient depending on how busy they are, although this is sometimes up for negotiation. Sylvia is a seasoned, no-nonsense nurse. When the charge nurse, Ivy, asks her to go to room 2 to give a RhoGAM shot, Sylvia does not hesitate or try to negotiate her way out of this task, something some nurses routinely do. She finds that the unit has no shots and quickly makes her way to the several-minutes-away lab, which involves going down some stairs, around several corners, up some stairs, and around more corners before arriving at the lab. She verifies the patient's name and gets the shot from the attendant, and we make our way back to the unit, where she administers the shot and documents everything.

Further, nurses must personally stay up-to-date on protocols (which are constantly changing), and nurses often consult the protocol binder in anticipation of a patient they are being assigned or while caring for a patient. Competencies are also required once a year. This entails nurses doing online and live-station training to ensure they are current in their clinical knowledge. Some training can be done while on duty, if the nurse has time, or she may come in to do training during an on-call shift. I was in the hospital in January 2014 when nurses were completing online competencies on what was defined as a slow day. I was struck with how nurses had pages and pages of material to read before taking an online test. This structure almost promotes nurses' skimming the material and then taking the test, which can be retaken if an adequate score is not obtained. Reading the materials thoroughly would take quite a bit of time, and the nurses were doing this while also having to care for patients, hardly a system to promote nurses' taking the online competencies seriously. In addition, mandatory trainings are required when the hospital obtains new equipment. I attended mandatory training on how to use a transcutaneous bilirubinmeter (testing a baby's bilirubin by scanning his/her forehead) and on the Panda Warmer, an integrated infant incubator, warmer, and scale, which was being introduced in the ORs and NICU.

I would be remiss if I did not mention things nurses are asked to do that would seem to be totally outside of reasonable expected behavior. For example, in one of my observations, while preparing to administer an epidural to a labor patient, the anesthesiologist's cell phone rings with a text notification. His phone is in the front pant pocket of his scrubs. Julie is hanging a bag of fluid on the IV pole when he turns to her and demands that she grab his cell phone out of his pants pocket. She complies, deftly putting her hand in his front pocket, withdrawing the cell phone, and showing it to him. He nods and tells her to place the phone on the patient's table. I found this interaction almost unbelievable—that is, the idea of a nurse being asked to place her hand into a physician's front pants pocket to retrieve a phone—but when I relay this story to nurses and doctors, they are not surprised, saying that it is typical of the hierarchy between nurses and doctors. Another example of such behavior is that a very senior nurse told me she will not tolerate physicians yelling at her. Her articulation of this rule followed a more general discussion at the desk in which many nurses were discussing their frustration with physicians yelling at them when they call at night about a patient.

I have done my best to capture the tasks and complexity of an OB nurse's typical day caring for a laboring patient. There is much walking, charting, checking vitals, and dealing with beeping machines that goes on day after day. Some days are frantically busy with hardly a minute to eat even a snack, while other days are painfully slow. However, the definition of slow and busy changed over time, as I will discuss throughout the book.

Differences Pre- and Post-Axiom

Throughout the book, I draw a distinction in how the nurses are affected in what I call the "pre-Axiom" period and the "post-Axiom" period. The reader will recall that the Axiom merger was not implemented. Axiom pulled out of the deal in December 2014, reportedly because of stipulations the state put on other impending hospital mergers in the state. Yet the pre-Axiom period, although chaotic, was a time of anticipation and excitement for the hospital administrators and employees. Axiom was their "saving grace." When Axiom pulled out, the hospital was thrust again into even more uncertainty about its future. I suggest that these are conceptually different periods and treat them as such. Thus, in the following two chapters, I discuss and document the changing role of nurses during the pre- and post-Axiom periods. In order to substantiate how and why I see these periods as different, I end this chapter by noting several changes that are only apparent through the longitudinal observations I made at the hospital. I will draw these out more in the coming chapters, but I want to note them here so that they are apparent as one reads the book.

The Unit Became Exponentially Busier

Before Axiom pulled out of the acquisition deal, the unit was much less busy, even on days defined as busy. For example, in November 2013 I was in the hospital on a day that I recorded in my notes as seeming busy:

> A pediatrician is discharging patients [babies]. Lori mentions that she wants lactation to see a mom because the baby has lost 10 percent of its body weight. She wants the lactation consultant to see her first [before the pediatrician does] "to get us another room." This was the theme for the day—too many patients, not enough rooms.

In other words, Lori is hoping that a consultation with the lactation consultant to help the mom with nursing will dissuade the pediatrician from compelling the patient to stay another night at the hospital, thereby freeing up a room. Lori knows they need the room. My next note is that there are only four LDRP rooms open and no extended-stay rooms. It is a busy day. Having four LDRP rooms in the "post-Axiom world" would be a luxuriously slow day, and the slow day would be appreciated as a break from the common mayhem. This is how dramatic changes were in the unit.

In fact, *not* being busy was a perpetual concern before January 2015. Nurses commonly joked about my showing up on slow days. However, the joke also showed some anxiety the nurses had about not being busy. If the unit is not busy, nurses are often placed on call, and this affects their pay. During one of my observations in March 2014, the nurses told me how they had just had a month of really slow days with not a lot of births and that had put everyone on edge. I asked them why. One nurse says, "Well, you know, if we don't have enough people in the hospital, then we get put on call. And, the problem with being on call is that you are sent home effectively and only make seven dollars per hour." Further, the nurses tell me that they had attended meetings in which they were told that the low numbers were a problem. On this day in March 2014, the nurses are excited because the unit is busy and no one is being put on call. They are happy to be busy. The tone of the nurses is gleeful.

Fast-forward one year to March 2015, and "busy" was defined and thought about very differently. This changing definition contrasts with the "busy" unit before the Axiom deal fell apart and the new practices affiliated with Fuller Hospital. Part of the frustration for the nurses was that the unit was to have been renovated and additional LDRP rooms built before the new practices started deliveries at the hospital. However, this did not happen. This disjuncture is not missed by the nurses, who fully see the illogic of how this decision took place. Here Kerry expresses her frustration with the situation in our December 2015 interview:

> In the spring, we were told we were getting this group coming, and we were told we would be getting these rooms and the staffing, and we assumed we'd be getting the rooms and then the staffing and then the patients, but we got the patients, *without* the rooms and the staffing . . . And I think that was just really frustrating for everyone because we knew it was motivated by money, and it didn't have the best for the patients in mind. It wasn't about giving them the best, it was about money. And so, I think that was just a real frustration for a lot of us. Because when you think about it, it makes sense to hire staff and get rooms, and then have

more patients come to deliver vulnerable, small children, you know? Not, "Get a lot of new people, and have them deliver in closets until we can figure something else out," you know? It just didn't seem right.

Construction was put on hold when Axiom pulled out of the acquisition agreement. Cynthia, a unit administrator, told me that all meetings about the new construction ceased: "We stopped the meetings about it. We stopped everything. Everything just ground to a halt."

Jamie, a night nurse, tied the introduction of the new obstetrical practices to significant changes in her work life: "There was a huge boom . . . when they started. I mean, we're busy all the time. We used to have really dead [nights] . . . where you only had two mother-baby pairs on the floor. That doesn't happen to us anymore." Evelyn tells me in an April 2015 interview that when a nurse signs up for call, she will almost always be called into work, which leaves nurses working more hours than they bargained for:

> A lot of the nurses are saying [that] when you sign up for call, you might as well just expect that you're working it, because it's highly unlikely that they won't call you. . . . I mean we're all working a lot. There's a level of fatigue that comes with that, where you used to give up a few hours here and a few hours there occasionally. Now it's your thirty-two-hour position has turned into a thirty-six-to-forty-hour position, because you can pretty much count on the fact that you're going to be going in for your call.

Rachel describes the unit as "different":

> We're a very different unit than what we used to be. So, a lot of bigger hospitals, busier hospitals, . . . for every shift they have techs that maybe they can be stocking our ready rooms and stripping the rooms . . . I can't tell you how many times as charge nurse in a panic for a room I've gone in the room and stripped it all down, in addition to my assignment . . . for fear of having that patient who doesn't have a room, or having that delivery in a place that shouldn't be happening. . . . So, I feel like we're a different unit than when I first started here, and they've done really great things to get us more staff with the increased volume, but I think . . . still

other support staff as well [are needed]. . . . I used to not think . . . "What would we do if we had aides . . . or . . . techs? There'd be nothing for them to do." And now I think, "Oh, it'd be really great . . . to have someone to go throw the OR back together . . . or to go get the rooms ready, instead of having one of your nurses do that." . . . I think it's the unit, the unit is different. . . . The volume with the new [practice], it's a different unit.

Kerry tells me that in the summer of 2015, pressure to work extra shifts was at an extreme. She explains, "There [were] a lot of calls and texts this summer, a lot of these, 'We're desperate' . . . More so than, 'We're just short.' You know, but, 'We are desperate.'" Jamie also mentions this issue in an interview:

Everybody's posting on our little Facebook site we have that's strictly just for our nurses. . . . Most of the time it's "We have too many labors and not enough nurses, who wants to come to work?" That's what it's like every day, and you just ignore it because I can't go in there more. I don't wanna go in there more. It's like, you know, if I go in there the life is sucked out of me for twelve hours. I don't really wanna go in there on a different day. . . . Then you get the nursing staff, who some of them are very negative and some of them are like, for a while there, they were always mad at the people that wouldn't come in more. . . . You can't be mad at your peers for not filling the holes that management is not taking care of.

Unit revenues no doubt went up with the addition of the two new practices, and nurses reported to me that upper-level administrators routinely came by the unit in 2015 to tell them that they were the only hospital unit that was making money. They were proud of this but also found stressful the idea that their unit alone was keeping the hospital afloat. What they found with the extra babies that came with the new practices was that they were busy—too busy according to most nurses. They told me that it was "summer all year long," a nod to how the summer tended to have a higher number of babies born. I was told tales of women delivering vaginally in a cesarean recovery room or in a triage room, neither of which even has a bathroom. Busy was not having only *four* LDRP rooms like it was in the Pre-Axiom period; busy was having *no* LDRP rooms. During one of my observations in November 2015, a physician complained that her patient's vital signs had not been taken during the night shift. We learn this is because the unit was busy, really busy the night before. In other words, pre-Axiom, the nurses did not know busy, or at least not consistent busyness.

Further, it is not just nurses who are affected by the new practice and the hiring of new nurses. Administrators also have to deal with these changes. In April 2015 Cynthia told me how she was overwhelmed by her responsibilities:

> We had a serious safety event that happened in January while I was away, and, when I got back, I got hit with all of these new hires and all the responsibilities—the action plan for the state that we had to meet all these requirements. . . . And so, I've been, you know, actually I just feel like I'm just barely getting my head above water right now.

Equipment Is Forever Missing

I was struck by how often I went with nurses to look for missing equipment or to look for a replacement for broken equipment. Pauline, a unit administrator, told me in a May 2014 interview when discussing changes at the hospital, "I think the biggest barrier [to providing support to the nurses] is financial and all of the things that go along with financial . . . having times where you might not have . . . the best equipment." Problems with missing or inferior equipment became worse over time. Ashley, in a straightforward way, summarizes, "We constantly are missing equipment." The nurses also must deal with equipment that does not work, and this problem became worse as time went on.

In one of my observations in November 2015, Wendy is caring for a mother-baby pair and is getting inconsistent readings of the baby's blood sugar level. She tells other nurses at the front desk that one time she got thirty, which is too low, and another time she got forty-two, which is fine, and this is from the same blood sample. She concludes, "This is just unreliable. I don't want my kid to go to the NICU because my scanner doesn't work." She goes to the NICU to try another scanner. During this same observation, a physician finds that she cannot read a paper she prints with patient information. The secretary tells her that it is not a toner issue but a printer problem. The physician says, "Are you kidding me? I can't even read this."

Jamie, a seasoned nurse, overflowed with examples about missing equipment. It was clear in talking with her that what I was seeing was not unique to the nurses I followed. Missing equipment is a systemic problem affecting nurses' everyday working lives. Jamie explains:

> [Missing equipment/supplies] always seems to be the problem. . . . I'm in the OR, somebody drops the cord blood thing, and I go to find it and there aren't any more tubes . . . or you can't find [them]. I spend twenty more minutes running around the unit trying to find a red blood tube that we can put some cord blood in because there aren't any. Or, you know, you go in and there's no linens in the linen cart because nobody ordered it in the evenings. Or . . . you go to the placenta bucket place, and there's no placenta buckets. . . . We had two warmers out of commission. Well, I can't have that. I had to take a warmer out of the NICU because the bed part of it was broken. . . . I'm like well there's one in the nursery that's not being used. I'm going to have to take it because I don't have a room for the next patient who walks in at eight centimeters. . . . I had no IV pumps the other night. . . . So, I had to go into the room when the patient was sleeping. Take her pump, wipe it down, bring it to the room for the patient that went to the OR so that . . . the nurse who's taking care of that patient will then, at the end of her shift, . . . have to wipe it down, when she didn't need it anymore, and bring it back to her patient who's going to be induced in the morning. I mean . . . that's all you do all night long, is like rob Peter to pay Paul.

However, equipment failure and lack of equipment is not just an inconvenience. This can be a safety issue as well. Jamie goes on in her interview to give me an example of how financial constraints of the hospital have real effects on patients:

> I go in the other night, there's not enough equipment for all the patients that are in labor, and . . . the baby is delivered. I put the baby on the warmer . . . and all of a sudden, it [the warmer] starts screaming "system fail" . . . and the patient is looking at me. I'm like, "I'm really sorry. The baby is fine. It's

just screaming system fail." Well I don't even have another warmer to re-place it with, so I dry the baby off. I put it back on my mom's skin. I'm like, "Well, I guess I need to go figure something else [out]." . . . I didn't need to resuscitate the baby, thank God. It was fine. I just needed to pink it up a little bit and rub it off, dry it off, and clamp the cord, and I gave it back to the mother. But I'm like, "What am I supposed to do now?" . . . It's trouble-shooting. Why doesn't this piece of equipment work? Why won't this moni-tor hook up to our central monitoring system? Why is that cord broken? Why isn't this thing working? Why is there no computer that works in the triage room? How am I supposed to get the patient from downstairs in the ER, because I don't have another nurse to send downstairs, so I'm going to send the tech and hope to God she doesn't deliver in the wheelchair on the way up? . . . I feel like my job now is just putting out fires.

Patient Care Is Compromised

Nurses were also expected to have different responsibilities and different patient loads in the post-Axiom period. This included being assigned more mother-baby pairs. Rachel told me that at times nurses have been assigned five pairs to look after at one time, higher than is allowed per their professional guidelines and per hospital policy. A perhaps unrec-ognized issue, too, is that nurses may have even more than five pairs because they may be caring for patients *on top of those pairs* if another nurse has been called to the OR to scrub or circulate or if another nurse is taking a lunch break.

Nurses also told me that having two labor patients, a once unheard-of activity, was now common. Amanda and Tammy, nurses on the unit, explain:

> AMANDA: If we're short nurses, then you're going to get two labor patients. It's just one of those things.
> THERESA: Really? Even if [the patients] are [in] active [labor]?
> AMANDA: Yeah. I've had two active, yeah.
> THERESA: Have you?
> AMANDA: With an orientee. . . . That was bad. And they both got to fully dilated, too.
> THERESA: At a similar time?

AMANDA: Yeah.

TAMMY: At that point, if you had to push with one of them, you would have to have the charge nurse look after the other one.

Unit administrators knew these patient loads would be increased with the new practices. This new volume was expected. Unit administrator Anna tells me:

> [The nurses are] just starting to feel the impact now, 'cause summertime's really busy as far as people wanting to have babies in the summer, number one. . . . Now we have this new group, and then we have staff who are on vacation. . . . And then not only are your staff on vacation, the per diems [i.e., nurses who do not work on a set schedule but work shift to shift] that you use to backfill are also on vacation. . . . So, your pool of nurses is very slim at the busiest time of the year. So, I feel like that has really impacted sort of the feel of the unit. . . . That's been a difficult challenge.

According to Cynthia, another unit administrator, "We've been busting at the seams a good part of this year."

Lauren, a nurse on the unit, tells me that continuity of care is affected because she cannot, with any kind of regularity, have the same patient two days in a row. This could be a patient in labor for two days or a patient who delivers one day and needs postpartum care the next day. With so many more patients, this type of flexibility is now gone, Lauren tells me. Tammy also discussed this in her interview. She tells me, "When it gets crazy, like it will, . . . I [can't] split myself in all the different places if all the different babies [have] different issues, if our moms [have] different issues. You can't give them as much care as you'd normally give to them." Later in the interview Tammy continues with this theme. She tells me, "We like continuity here. . . . Now . . . you might have to dump 'em because you['ve] got to take a labor. . . . You try to tie 'em up with a bow as best you can, and then you move on, which a lot of us don't like. We like being able to spend time with the patient."

There Are Lots of New Nurses

This busyness and resulting stress on nurses led to the unit administrators' hiring more nurses. However, this was not the only reason new nurses were hired. The hiring of new nurses was also due to experienced nurses quitting and taking jobs in other hospitals or in other segments of the health-care industry. In my notes from November 16, 2015, I wrote, upon arriving at the unit, "Everyone is new." Hiring so many new nurses had ramifications. Nurses complained to me that they often did not know they had a nurse orientee until she showed up. They said they handled it but would like some warning. Some nurses said this was a scheduling issue, but, regardless, it was clear that having so many orientees was problematic. I documented in my notes that when new nurses are being oriented, patient care suffers. The orientees are so focused on learning the documentation system that they do not always hear what patients are saying to them or even notice when the patient is having a contraction. Consequently, more experienced nurses became tired of new nurses.

I interviewed Cynthia, a unit administrator, in December 2015, a time of continued uncertainty and frustration. I questioned her about the nurses' increased work of orienting new nurses and teaching residents and student nurses. She told me that nurses were being asked to do more and more:

> I see what these wonderful nurses are trying to accomplish and so much is being put on them. . . . It's so much being asked of them these days that has not been asked before. . . . When I first got here, I will never forget someone saying . . . "Well, the wonderful thing about education here at DHN is . . . when we roll something new out and the staff have something new that they have to do, . . . we're going to take something away. . . . We'll make it fair." . . . I haven't seen anything taken away yet. No, not even once. We just pile it on, and pile it on, and pile it on and expect them to take it.

New nurses mean that the current nurses must train them. Nurses recognize having so much teaching to do as a burden and not consistent with what they viewed as their role. Jennifer told me, "It's med students, residents, nursing students, and orientees. You've got it all. And the nursing students ask a lot of questions. . . . And, you know, I never said I wanted to be a teacher. . . . So that's another job." When I asked about how this had changed, she told me that orientees used to be "few and far between" and that there are now more nursing students. She attributed more nursing students to more patients because the supervisors take students to hospitals where deliveries are likely.

Nurses' frustration came through to the orientees. Cynthia, a unit administrator, described how having so many new nurses causes stress and frustration on the unit, and how some of the new nurses complained to her that they did not feel welcome in the unit:

> We have hired quite a few new people, and so everyone was a little worried about that. It has been a little bit of a challenge with hiring that many people all at once. There [have] been some uncomfortable moments. We had some . . . new hires in my office saying "I don't feel welcome; I don't feel wanted." But, you know, there has been a little bit higher level of stress. . . . We have had more patients. We have been busier since the new practices started. . . . We have been . . . booming, booming busy and had 3 West open and . . . it's been crazy, and people are stressed. And then when you say, "Okay, now I have three orientees who need to go with nurses and somebody needs to precept them." . . . Everybody is like, "No! No! No!" . . . And they can sometimes be rude to these poor new people who are just trying to learn and . . . they're just coming into this situation. They don't know. So, it's been a little bit of a challenge.

The unit was a more relaxed place to work pre-Axiom. There was missing equipment, no doubt, and that hampered patient care. Yet the slower pace and preponderance of more seasoned nurses gave it a feeling of a stable and collegial place to work. This all changed. For example, Jennifer tells me about her friendly relationship with another nurse: "We have to get together outside of work, even though we work together, because we both have orientees all the time, we have another person right there . . . So, it wasn't fun anymore to come [to work]." As Jennifer's words indicate, when Axiom pulled out, things changed. Nurses became downtrodden and many left. I witnessed much more arguing, petty talk about one another, and sometimes crying. I sensed that there had been a fundamental transformation in terms of workplace for the nurses. I saw frustration grow over time, especially after the new practices were added. Jamie told me in a September 2015 interview how she saw discord in the unit and that nurses are looking for employment elsewhere:

> So, it becomes this nasty, also internal, negative environment where people are being mean to each other. . . . I go in. I do my job. I don't work a ton of extra. I can get my smile on. I mean I can do all this stuff, but . . . people are just gonna disappear, like pretty soon we aren't going to have anyone working here anymore.

After March 2015, it was not uncommon in my observations to see nurses, especially charge nurses, in tears, something I never saw before Axiom pulled out of the acquisition. The frustration and anger was present in the unit every time I observed in the post-Axiom period.

These concerns were at an alarming level during my observation period in November 2015, during which time employee forums were held. Although nurses encouraged me to attend, and I am sure I would have learned quite a lot, my IRB-approved project did not extend to employee forums. I did learn from the nurses about what happened at the forums. Nurses who stayed with the old pension system had been promised that the hospital would contribute to it by the end of December 2015. A nurse showed me an email that was distributed by the hospital administration earlier in the year indicating this. At the forum, the administration announced that they were not going to make the promised pension contribution. In talking about the forum, I learned, too, that OR nurses had been laid off the week before. Although there had been a rumor that nurses from the OB unit would be laid off, this fear had not come to pass.

As another indication of the fun being taken out of work, nurses no longer left the floor to go to nearby shops, such as Starbucks or Dunkin' Donuts, for coffee for themselves and their coworkers. Or, if not to leave the hospital, nurses would go to the gift shop for some candy or mints. Although these types of outings or errands did not totally stop, they had curtailed quite a bit, such that by November 2015, even when a nurse went out of the hospital for lunch when she was clocked out, the other nurses were a bit shocked. They were so busy, it was hard to imagine nurses leaving, even for a few minutes and while on their own time.

Staff Support Was Cut

Support staff was cut back over the time period I studied the hospital. This was particularly apparent with custodians and secretaries. I am not able to get exact numbers, but I can say that when I observed the hospital before Axiom pulled out of the acquisition, I saw custodians all the time. I was struck how nurses often ignored the custodian as she used a cloth to wipe the phones and desk counter where they worked. They would just wheel their chairs back to give her access to the counter. She also swept around their feet. This was routine and happened in nearly every observation I made. At other times, there were two or three custodians on the floor mopping and buffing the hall floors. This type of diligent and routine cleaning was uncommon after Axiom pulled out. The one custodian I typically saw on the floor during any one of my observational periods was clearly taxed with duties, and I hardly ever saw her cleaning the front desk. In fact, when I conducted observations over a week in November 2015, I wrote in my notes, "I've been here for a whole week, long day and evening shifts and sometimes into the night shifts. There has not been one custodian come behind the desk to clean." In my last observation in June 2016 I actually saw dust balls and trash on the floor throughout the hallways and behind the desk.

Another indication that hospital administrators have cut custodial staff hours is that sharps containers (where used syringes are safely deposited) were full throughout the unit during an observation in November 2015. The NICU's containers were overflowing, and the secretary called and asked for them to be changed. Later, an anesthesiologist comes out of room with a used syringe in hand and asks where to find a sharps container that is not full. The nurses tell him the number of a room in which they think he'll be able to find a sharps container. I had not previously observed any issue with the sharps containers being full.

Another example of outcomes of custodial cuts comes from a November 2015 observation. I accompanied Evelyn into a triage room, where she was evaluating a patient who complained of cramps and diarrhea and who, upon examination, had alarmingly high blood pressure. After evaluating the patient, Evelyn noticed a used speculum (a tool used to widen a woman's vagina for a cervical exam) sitting on top of the fetal heart monitor. She put on gloves, picked it up while wearing a disgusted face, and took it out of the room. I accompanied her. She told me she could not believe she had found a used speculum in a "clean" triage room. She took it to the trash room, sprayed it with disinfectant, and put it in a bag to be cleaned. This is an indication of what happens when custodial staff is cut and cleaning gets done too quickly.

The hours of other support staff were also cut. Secretarial hours were reduced in the fall of 2015 across the entire hospital. This had a negative effect on nurses, who must pick up secretarial tasks that still need to be performed. I saw this happen numerous times in my observations after the hour cut. Lauren, a nurse in the unit, told me in a November 2015 interview, when I asked how she was being affected by changes going on in the hospital:

> Nursing staff is being affected by our secretaries getting a cut in their hours, because they do things for us that we just know are going to be done and taken care of. And then we have to stop and do it. . . . Yes, all of us nurses know how . . . to put together a chart. We know how to do X, Y, or Z. But it's so much easier for us to just pay attention to our patient and not have to worry about coming to the desk and printing off the chart, blah, blah, blah. . . . Secretaries . . . know about the supplies. They know where they are and when we're low on them. . . . It's just more and more and more on our plate without any . . . recognition as we have gotten increasingly busier with our . . . patient . . . level.

This problem with cutting the hours of support staff is that the consequences extend to other support staff as well. I interviewed a nurse with over twenty-five years of experience, Carolyn, and asked her about missing equipment and supplies. She tied it to staff cuts at the hospital: "When they reduce their staff by half downstairs, of course we're going to feel some effect of it."

Patient Safety Was Compromised

There is other evidence of how crisis affects patient care. External groups have penalized the hospital for its care of patients. For example, the Leapfrog Group awarded the hospital a grade of D on patient safety in the spring of 2016.[9] Hospitals that are rated D have a 50 percent higher risk of avoidable death than do hospitals that are rated A. This score is a slip for Fuller, which received a C rating in 2013, 2014, and 2015. Further, Fuller was penalized in 2015 and 2016 by CMS (Centers for Medicare and Medicaid Services) for having a higher than expected hospital acquired infection rate, a concerning measure in terms of patient safety. This rating led to the hospital's losing 1 percent of its Medicare payments, quite a blow to an already struggling institution.

I share here a specific example of change that affected patient safety. In my observation period at the hospital in November 2015, there had been three post-surgery cesarean infections in a short span, and the number had reached eleven by June 2016. Doctors and nurses speculated about what was causing this. To deal with the spike, two new protocols were introduced. The first protocol I mentioned above, that of requiring nurses to wear hospital-laundered scrubs. The second protocol was for nurses to wash women's abdomens before surgery to make sure they were as sterile as possible. Nurses were frustrated with this protocol and thought that women would prefer to wash themselves. Yet, when I interviewed a unit administrator in December 2015 about this spike in infections, she told me that the infection outbreak might actually be due to custodial cutbacks, which neither scrubs nor a new abdomen-washing practice would solve:

> We've had more post-c-section infections than we would want to see in a certain period of time. . . . It could be that we have something going on that we need to address to make sure that our sterility is absolutely perfect in our ORs. And one of those things has to do with the cleaning of our ORs. . . . We had . . . the head of the environmental services department in that meeting saying "Well . . . our staffing has been cut . . . There's only two people on at night and . . . I don't think we could manage to get, you know, [we're] supposed to be doing this [OR cleaning] every twenty-four hours, and . . . we just don't have enough people to do it.

The post-cesarean infection problem had not been solved as of June 2016, six months after being identified.

Bolstering Cynthia's analysis that custodial cuts may be at the root of the high post-cesarean infection rate in the hospital, it came out during my June 2016 observations that custodians had been told to "terminally" clean the OR after each cesarean and to sign off that they had done so. The catch: they are not really doing a "terminal" clean, which takes hours due to the necessity of cleaning the ceilings and walls. A custodian in the unit was concerned because her boss had told her to sign off on terminal cleaning the OR when she had not in fact terminally cleaned it. She told one of the OB unit administrators that she did not know what to do. The unit administrator told her not to sign off on a terminal clean and that she would call the custodian's boss. No doubt this mandate was put in place to deal with the post-cesarean infection rate, but it shows the concerning lack of resources in the hospital and how different units are passing the buck—or, in an even more concerning interpretation, how they are deceiving other units to avoid being blamed for a problem.

Surprisingly, New Equipment Was Purchased

Finally, the one change that benefited nurses was that having the new practices gave the nurse manager increased leverage to request new positions and more equipment—thermometers, spotlights, and a few new fetal monitors. Further, as will be seen in coming chapters, a particularly vexing problem for nurses was not having thermometers and blood pressure cuffs in every room. That problem was solved in November 2015 when, seemingly overnight, thermometers were indeed placed in every room. One nurse started to wheel a thermometer cart toward a room one day in late November 2015. The secretary stopped her and told her that there were now thermometers in every room, to which she replied, "Thermometers in every room? Really?" However, this was not a perfect arrangement because they were affixed to the wall by the head of the bed and had a short cord, meaning that if the patient strayed far from the bed, the nurse had a hard time using the thermometer. Also, the thermometer did not reach the crib. The nurses were happy with the new equipment but frustrated that they had not been asked about how they used the thermometer and where in the room it should be placed. But, still, this is a sign of progress. Thus, the new practices did benefit the nurses in some ways. A funny anecdote I will share concerns physicians' and nurses' jokes about a new tub in the tub room that lights up in different colors. A physician says incredulously, "There's no money, but we have a tub with lights." A nurse responds, "It was probably the only one left and on clearance."

Conclusion

Nurses have a complex job, and that job was made more difficult over the three years I conducted observations. The hospital administrators strive to deal with changes coming from the external environment, but nurses are the ones who must deal with those changes most directly in terms of patient care. However, it should be clear that hospital administrators made decisions about how to handle changes imposed on them from national and state-level policies. Organizational theory predicts that decisions will be made to deal with changes in the political environment, and the unit that most controls such decisions is that unit which deals most directly with the uncertainty.[10] Thus, it is clear from theory that one would expect the CEO and board of trustees, individuals who deal with the hospital finances, to make decisions. However, the decisions they made created irrationalities within the hospital that directly affected nurses, as well as physicians and hospital staff, and made patient care less safe.

PART II

Nursing and Organizational Change

3

Patient-Oriented Nurses

> A less-seasoned nurse would have let that patient have a c-section. There are also some older nurses who would have let the patient have a c-section. (Kim)

Kim, a nurse with close to ten years' experience, tells me this over lunch about an hour after her patient pushed for three hours until finally delivering her baby vaginally. Kim is hungry and exhausted. Pushing is not only taxing for patients but for nurses, too. During the patient's three hours of pushing, Kim constantly changed the patient's position—squatting bar, hands and knees, sitting back and pulling on a sheet—until, finally, the baby was born vaginally. It was clearly a tight fit—the baby's head was shaped like a pointed cone. What I contend is that it is not being a more- or less-seasoned nurse that led Kim to help this woman attain a vaginal birth. Rather, it is her patient orientation. Patient-oriented nurses define patient care as their primary goal. They complete their paperwork, but the paperwork is not central to their identity or job. Instead, they focus on making sure the patient's experience is as good as it can be and is as close as possible to her stated wishes for her labor and birth.[1]

Kim used her knowledge and bag of tricks throughout the patient's labor to try to facilitate a vaginal birth. Kim not only helped the patient change position to encourage cervical dilation, she also held off the physician who was all too willing to step in with a surgical delivery (i.e., a cesarean). The patient pushed for an extended time, and in such a situation physicians often become impatient. They may worry about spending too much time on the labor of one patient and also that the baby might not fit through the woman's birth canal, a condition called cephalopelvic disproportion (CPD). How long a woman should "be allowed" to push is contentious and has been a point of considerable debate in public health discussions focusing on increasing a woman's likelihood of

vaginal delivery.[2] One of the few randomized controlled trials to examine how pushing time affects birth outcomes found that women who are
allowed prolonged time to push compared to women who are not have a
50 percent reduction in their likelihood of a cesarean without increasing
maternal or neonatal morbidity (i.e., injury).[3]

After the patient has been pushing for a little over an hour, Kim sees
the physician charting at the front desk. Kim had just put the patient
on her hands and knees because they have figured out that the baby is
coming out face up (posterior) and the hands-and-knees position may
spin the baby face down (anterior), an easier position for a baby to be
born vaginally. The physician tells Kim that the baby is not moving. Kim
replies in a friendly way, "She's doing everything I ask, and her temperature is still fine." They are watching the patient's temperature because her
amniotic sac is ruptured, which increases the chance of uterine infection. Kim is asserting in a friendly way that the patient has time—there
is no rush. The physician does not respond. About thirty minutes later
she again advocates for the patient when the physician is in the room
to check the patient's progress by putting her gloved fingers inside the
woman's vagina as she pushes. The patient pushes, and Kim says, "It
looks like the baby came down." I write in my notes that she is trying
hard to convince the physician of the patient's progress. The physician
responds, "A little bit."

Two more incidences of Kim's advocacy are worth mentioning.
Nearly three hours into pushing, just as the physician enters the room,
the father of the baby says that his wife is worried she is not big enough
for the baby to get through her birth canal. Kim quickly responds with
a smile, "Everything looks good. Let me worry about that. Now, let's
show [the physician] what you've done." Finally, a full three hours after
the patient started pushing, the physician asks Kim how long the patient
has been pushing. Kim looks at the charts and says, "A little over two
hours," a deliberate deception. It is hard to know if Kim's advocacy led
to a vaginal birth, but the patient delivered vaginally just twenty minutes
after her white lie.

Notice in this observation how Kim's care is intensive and her advocacy is essential. Part of her success is likely due to her having only one
patient to manage. She is not asked to take a mother-baby pair (or two)
or even a triage patient. This is the pre-Axiom world. I cannot write

about Kim after the Axiom acquisition offer fell apart. She left her job at Fuller Hospital in December 2013 to be a nurse at a clinic specializing in women's health. It is hard to know if she left because of the uncertainty caused by financial troubles in the hospital, but given that her departure came at the start of a steady flow of nurses leaving the hospital, it is not hard to imagine that this may have had some effect.

This chapter highlights nurses who are patient oriented in my categorization. Patient-oriented nurses put front and center helping patients attain the birth they want, or at least getting them as close to that ideal as possible. They spend time with patients and embody what would be commonly defined as the nurturing behavior that is stereotypically associated with the nursing occupation. Nurturing behavior is also associated with women and is gendered in that way to the extent that all nurses in this unit are female. In other words, patients value these nurses' behavior perhaps because it aligns well with normative behavior expected of women. As a result, social rewards abound for such nurses. I highlight patient-oriented nurses in this chapter, focusing on how different the time before Axiom rescinded its acquisition offer to Fuller (December 2014) was from the time after (January 2015 and later). I show how conditions changed dramatically, not only for the nurses, but for the patients, too.

Rachel

When I interviewed Rachel in the summer of 2015, she had been a nurse for more than ten years. She described to me how she entered the nursing field. First, she applied to college to be an education major because she thought that she wanted to be a teacher. However, she changed her mind just before starting classes her freshman year. She recalls:

> Visiting people in the hospital, I always really kind of liked to be there, whether it was babies, or grandparents, or whatever. And initially when I was going to school I kept telling everybody that I wanted to be a teacher, because I was afraid to say that I wanted to be a nurse.

I asked her why she was afraid to say she wanted to be a nurse. She answered:

I don't know. . . . It was right before there was like . . . jobs for everybody as a nurse. I was sitting with my dad at dinner one night, and I'm like, "I don't think I'm going to be a teacher. I think I want to be a nurse." And he said, "Well, call right now. Call the school. Change your major."

She did just that and obtained a four-year nursing degree.

Nurses, just like doctors, specialize in a given area. I asked Rachel how she came to become an OB nurse. She told me that she knew right out of college she wanted to be an OB nurse. However, she worked for two years in a med-surg (medical-surgical) unit "to get my feet wet" and also because they offered her a job—she worked on the unit when she was in college as a summer nursing extern.[4] When a job opened in the neonatal intensive care unit at Fuller Hospital, she jumped. She tells me, "I kind of selfishly started here in the NICU . . . because I wanted to be in OB." Because the NICU is right next to the OB unit, she knew that she could likely transition from NICU to OB in the future. When I ask Rachel what she does to support patients, she says, "I think it's not being afraid to be a patient advocate, not being afraid to speak up and get the backlash from the doctor or the anesthesiologist . . . I think that's my biggest thing, and also a big thing for me is to treat others as I'd like to be treated." Notice how Rachel emphasizes how she treats and cares for patients and how advocacy is central to what she does as a nurse. She treats patients like she would like to be treated. This type of overtly caring personality and feeling that advocacy is a responsibility is typical of patient-oriented nurses. In an interview, Rachel describes a situation in which she advocated for a patient:

There's a particular doctor . . . who is very quick to intervene . . . or to want to do this or want to do that, [who] maybe could potentially say prematurely, "She's going to need a c-section." I remember, maybe it was about a year . . . and a half ago, I told him to go get lunch, or maybe to take a walk or something because he was thinking that she was going to have a c-section. . . . So, I said, "We need more time, it's going to happen." . . . So then [when he came back], she was fully dilated, we pushed, and we had a baby.

This type of advocacy is much more common among patient-oriented nurses, perhaps because they spend more time trying to understand what the patient wants.

Rachel Pre-Axiom

Rachel is a nurse who not only suggests that she espouses the golden rule of caring for patients but who embraces such a philosophy in her care. I share two observations of Rachel in the period before Axiom's acquisition of Fuller Hospital fell apart. I shared briefly from one of these observations in the book's introductory chapter that involved Rachel's care of a patient attempting a VBAC. I give more detail about that observation here. I also draw from my observation of Rachel's care of a patient being induced for chronic hypertension (high blood pressure).

Rachel cared for the VBAC patient in a July 2013 observation. The patient had planned a repeat cesarean but, upon arriving at the hospital, decided to attempt a vaginal delivery. Contextualization of this decision is important. Of the four OB practices that oversaw deliveries at this hospital in 2013, she was a patient of the practice *least* supportive of VBAC. Rachel knew this and, in fact, discussed it with me, telling me that the practice and the particular doctor on call for the practice were "very conservative" (conservative in this context means being very cautious about VBAC risks). The second observation is from November 2013, in which a patient is being induced at thirty-nine weeks because she has chronic hypertension. This is the patient's first pregnancy and birth, and her cervix is not "ready" (i.e., it is thick and closed). Such patients have a 50 percent chance of cesarean.[5] Rachel cares for the patient the morning after she had come to the hospital for an induction.[6] For both of these observations, Rachel was assigned only one patient for whom to care. This was typical in the pre-Axiom period.

I turn first to Rachel's care of the VBAC patient. The physician's conservative orientation around VBAC attempts comes out in her hesitance to use Pitocin in the care of a woman who had a previous cesarean. This is likely because the physician is concerned about the potential liability risk of using Pitocin to augment the contractions of a VBAC patient.[7] The patient's uterus might rupture (a very slight but serious risk for a woman laboring after having a cesarean), which may be more likely to happen with Pitocin augmentation.[8] In such a case, if there were a negative maternal or fetal outcome, the patient would most likely file a malpractice lawsuit against the physician. The patient asks Rachel whether she will be given Pitocin to make her contractions stronger. Rachel tells the patient that it depends on the doctor because doctors have different views on whether Pitocin should be given to VBAC patients. What she does not tell the patient is something she has already told me, that this doctor will likely not allow Pitocin. What Rachel does say to the patient is "It's good for you to be in labor either way. The baby will absorb some of the amniotic fluid. It is good for both of you to do some laboring." This is her way, by using positive language, of mediating what she knows about the physician and what the patient is asking for in care.

There are several instances throughout the day that make it clear how Rachel balances the conservative view of the physician and the wishes of the patient. She hooks the patient up to a telemetry unit to monitor the fetal heartbeat, which allows the patient to walk while still being monitored. Some nurses will have a patient stay in bed to monitor the fetal heartbeat, but Rachel not only suggests a telemetry unit but also makes sure her patient has one that reliably works. There is often competition over such units, to the extent that sometimes nurses will preemptively take a working telemetry unit into a patient's room before the patient needs it just to be sure it will be available when the patient wants to walk. Another example of how Rachel tries to facilitate a vaginal birth is that she encourages the patient to move around: "Sit in the rocking chair, walk the halls, lie down. Do whatever feels good," she tells the patient. Rachel encourages movement because she knows that movement helps labor progress. Rachel also suggests using a birth ball or peanut ball, both tools to help open a woman's pelvis in labor. Rachel tells the patient that, if she becomes tired, Rachel can put the peanut between the patient's legs and help her roll from side to side, even if the patient has an epidural.

Rachel goes to the patient's room many times to adjust the fetal heart monitor. This is something nurses spend much time doing. Fetuses move during labor, and finding their heartbeats can be difficult. This is especially the case if the woman is moving or walking in labor and/or if the patient is obese. I have written before about the lack of reliability of continuous fetal heart monitoring in terms of its ability to prevent bad birth outcomes, and this truth is still evident in literature on the fetal monitor.[9] In fact, the continuous use of fetal heart monitors is not linked to improved fetal outcomes but, paradoxically, is linked to a greater likelihood of cesarean, which puts a woman at higher risk of complications.[10] However, in many instances, protocol dictates continuous monitoring, such as when Pitocin is used, when the patient has an epidural, or, in this case, when the patient is attempting a VBAC. Because most patients meet one of the first two criteria, most are continuously monitored, and even those who do not meet the criteria will often be continuously monitored unless they specifically request intermittent monitoring. One trick nurses use when the monitor does not consistently pick up the fetal heartbeat is to put a coin under the monitoring belt where the device is tracking the fetal heart rate. Doing so gives the heart rate something hard to contact and sometimes leads to monitoring the fetal heartbeat more easily. Some nurses routinely keep a coin in the pocket of their scrubs for such an occasion. Rachel does not use a coin but rather spends much time in the patient's room adjusting the monitor, a more time-intensive way to deal with the problem. Yet she never shows any frustration with the situation.

Rachel's care of the induction patient corroborates her patient orientation. Rachel does something with this patient that I never saw another nurse do: she gives the patient some control over how quickly to increase Pitocin. Standard protocol in this OB unit is to increase Pitocin by two milliunits every thirty minutes. This is done until the patient reaches a protocol-defined maximum dose of twenty milliunits or until the patient has "adequate contractions," whichever comes first. When Rachel goes into the room thirty minutes after starting Pitocin, she gives the patient a choice about whether to go up one or two milliunits. Below is an excerpt from my notes:

> She tells them [the patient and her partner] that protocol is to go up on the Pitocin by two, but they can choose to go up by one. She asks the patient if she would like her to go up by two or one. The patient asks, "Can you turn it down?" Rachel tells her that they turn it down if they have too much. She says going up one or two is usually a nursing judgment. The patient asks, "Should I go up by two?" Rachel says, "At this point, that is acceptable. Is everyone on board? The goal is a happy mama, happy baby." She turns the Pitocin up two units.

She likely gave the patient the choice of how much to increase Pitocin because the patient's partner is quite controlling. He had very specific ideas about how labor should be (e.g., he did not want his partner to have an epidural) and was also assertive about other issues (e.g., Where can he recycle his Gatorade bottle NOW?). She is trying to help him (and the patient) be in control, and turning up the Pitocin by one or two milliunits likely would not make much of a difference in the patient's outcome.

Similar to her care of the VBAC patient, Rachel also repeatedly offers to get the birth ball for this patient, telling her that it might ease her discomfort. On her third offer, Rachel says, "Some love it; some hate it. You won't know until you try it." With this encouragement, Rachel leaves to get a birth ball for the patient. This example is interesting because not all nurses offer such tools without a request from the patient. This is an example of Rachel's being empathetic toward the patient, pulling out tricks from her knowledge base of how to facilitate a vaginal birth, which is the patient's stated goal.

The other practice Rachel uses is one that most patient-oriented nurses use—touch. Patient-oriented nurses typically feel a woman's abdomen when they want to know something about the strength of contractions. Process-oriented nurses tend to rely on the feedback of the contraction monitor attached to the woman. Rachel gives me a primer on how to tell contraction strength: feel your nose—not a strong contraction; feel your chin—a stronger contraction; feel your forehead—strong contraction. Feeling one's own face in this way indicates what a woman's uterus feels like with external palpation at different stages of labor. She uses touch to gauge contractions for both patients I highlight—the VBAC patient and induction patient. With the induction patient, Rachel tries to find the contractions so that she can adjust the monitor. When she is successful, she tells the patient, "Thank you for letting me feel!"

Rachel also tries her best to support patients' family and friends. For both patients, she points out that the chair next to the window folds out into a bed, demonstrating how this works. She makes sure to tell the family that there are extra sheets in the cabinet for the bed. She also tells the induction patient's partner that she left the food order in the patient's record (i.e., an order that gives permission for the cafeteria to prepare food for the patient). She tells him, "Obviously, she won't be eating, but *you* could order something *for her*," implying with her words and body language that he could eat the food ordered for the patient. She says, "This is a long day for you, too." Other, more process-oriented nurses simply tell the patient's partner that the cafeteria is on the first floor and closes at five o'clock.

It is also important to note that Rachel has fun at work. When she is at the desk while her patient walks the hall, she and the other nurses discuss vacations, family events, and kids. One sunny Friday, the nurses are sitting at the front desk chatting. Rain is predicted for the next day when one of the nurses has an outdoor birthday party scheduled for her young daughter. The nurses at the desk all give her advice, including holding the birthday party in her garage. In other words, the nurses have time and inclination to chat about their lives. My impression during this pre-Axiom observation is that they are enjoying themselves and that this would be a fun place to work.

Rachel Post-Axiom

To illustrate the differences from my earlier observations of Rachel before Axiom withdrew its acquisition offer to my observations after Axiom withdrew its offer, I draw first on the interview with Rachel in June 2015, after Axiom's withdrawal and not long after Waranoke's acquisition attempt was announced. Rachel tells me, "We're just so busy all the time . . . [This means,] depending on the busyness . . . not maybe sometimes being able to spend as much time with our patients as we would like to, depending on our assignment . . . I think it's more of the postpartum stuff." I followed up by inquiring about what she means by postpartum stuff. She tells me:

> I feel like if you have three, four, sometimes five pairs, if it's a really busy day . . . sometimes it happens . . . if you have a bunch of labors coming in, and your hands are tied . . . it can . . . impact patient care, number one, and number two . . . we have this unit, and we have 3 West, so a lot of times . . . if we have nurses coming in to help out, patients don't love having to go there, and they also don't love having maybe . . . four different nurses for only three- to four-hour periods.

Rachel is not just identifying a luxury the nurses once had of caring for no more than two mother-baby pairs. The Association of Women's Health, Obstetric and Neonatal Nurses (AWHONN) recommends that a nurse-to-patient ratio for healthy mother-baby pairs should be no more than one to three. In other words, caring for four or five pairs is outside the recommended guidelines. Further, the guidelines suggest a lower ratio when a cesarean is involved, if the woman is receiving magnesium sulfate during the postpartum period, and/or if the woman is a first-time mother.[11]

Rachel explained that part of the high assignment level is due to the hospital's opening 3 West as an overflow postpartum unit. As explained in chapter 1, this unit is in the hospital, but on a different floor and in a different wing. One registered nurse must be assigned to 3 West at all times, and she comes from the nurses on the unit. In other words, the unit loses a nurse when 3 West is open, meaning that the nurses assigned to mother-baby pairs have a higher assignment. Recall that 3 West is *only* open when the unit is full, a contradiction that most affects nurses assigned to mother-baby pairs. Opening 3 West as an overflow postpartum unit is no doubt due to the new practices bringing more births to the hospital, making the OB unit busy all the time. Rachel says, "We've always had spurts of busyness. Maybe we'll have a week here or there where it's like that [busy], but it wasn't consistently like that."

Rachel also indicates why being charge nurse is more stressful in the post-Axiom world. Charge nurses are responsible for making sure that an OR is ready at all times and that rooms are ready for patients. If the charge nurses are stressed, it is an indication of endemic stress because they are the most experienced and seasoned nurses. Let me share examples from Rachel about the accentuated stress of being in charge, something I discussed in chapter 2. One of my observations in November 2015 was during a week in which Rachel had been in charge for nearly all her shifts over the previous week. This frequency of being in charge took a toll on her. Just after her shift starts, it becomes apparent that being in charge is frustrating. She says, "I don't like being in charge because I've been in charge a lot." She sighs and, in her typical way of helping out, says that she can triage a "thirty-three weeker" who is coming in. She tells the other nurses, "I just need to go to talk to the section first."

Her day does not get any easier. The unit is busy, and rooms are scarce. Patients need to be transferred to 3 West. However, the nurse manager is nowhere to be found, and the nurses need a supervisor to approve the transfer. One nurse says, "We haven't even seen [the nurse manager]. Where is [the nurse manager]?" I had noticed earlier in the day a sign on the nurse manager's office door indicating that she was out for bereavement for three days, although perhaps nurses had not been notified or had missed an email notification. In order to transfer patients in the nurse manager's absence, Rachel has to make several phone calls to obtain the required approval.

The busyness of the day continues, with another indication being the frustration nurses have with a patient sent to the hospital for the nurses to rule out labor. The patient thinks her water has broken, but, using a simple test that can be performed in a physician's office, the nurse finds it has not. The nurses are frustrated that the patient takes a room when they are short on rooms, a frustration I had not seen in earlier observations. Women often come to the hospital thinking they have broken their water but, in fact, have not. The difference in how such patients are perceived in the post-Axiom world is striking.

Shortly afterward, another rule-out-labor patient arrives. Rachel finds Evelyn in room 4 and tells her that she's assigning her the triage patient coming in. Evelyn tells Rachel that she already has "done" one of this doctor's patients (this is a doctor reviled by the nurses). Evelyn continues, "I can't do another." Rachel, a generally calm, go-with-the-flow nurse, says in only a half-joking manner, "Do you want to do charge instead?" Evelyn emphatically says no. The discussion ends abruptly—no laughter, no more words. Tension is high. Evelyn relents and agrees to take the patient even though she is caring for a patient just out of a cesarean.

Ten minutes later a doctor calls about a postpartum hypertensive patient. He wants to admit the patient in the unit. Rachel is all business and says:

> We only have one labor room and one triage room. And, if the patient comes in, they're probably going to have to take the triage room because I can't take my last labor room for that patient. So, if you want them to come here, you can, or they can maybe go to the emergency department.

Although the words do not sound harsh, nurses rarely tell physicians directly that a patient cannot come in. These words take a great deal of courage from Rachel, and other nurses at the desk offer support, telling Rachel that she did the right thing. In fact, the patient does end up going directly to the ER and does not come to the OB unit.

Having solved this crisis, Rachel stands up and says, "Maybe the third time is a charm. I need to discharge room 5. Wish me luck." Rachel, even though she is in charge, has a patient assignment, but it is clear that her charge duties do not leave her time to do what she needs to do for this patient—get her discharged. One of the nurses at the desk asks Rachel if she would like her to do the discharge. Rachel replies, "No, no, I'm going to do it. I just haven't had time because I keep getting interrupted." She goes into room 5. At the same time, the expected triage patient shows up. A tech, who only recently joined the staff, is filling in temporarily as the secretary (in addition to her tech duties). She asks me whether Rachel has assigned someone to the triage patient. I know she has assigned Evelyn, and I tell her so.[12] The problem: Evelyn is nowhere to be found. The tech takes the patient to the triage room and comes back to the front desk. She tells the nurses there, "I gave her a gown and a band. Was that everything I was supposed to do?" They tell her, "Yes! Perfect!" Of course, the tech has not been trained on admissions and is just helping out, which explains her uncertainty as to what she should have done. The tech then asks me if I know where Rachel is. I tell her that I think room 5, but, when the tech checks room 5, Rachel is not there. She goes to look for Rachel *and* Evelyn. She finds Evelyn coming from the back hall toward the break room with her orientee, both holding trays from the cafeteria. Evelyn is frustrated when the tech tells her she just put the triage patient in a room. She tells the tech that Rachel knew she was going to eat and that she would not be able to take the triage patient until 2:00 (it is now about 1:40). She is frustrated and angry, but leaves her food in the break room and goes to the triage room to see about the patient. This observation is an indication of how crazy the unit had become. Evelyn is angry with Rachel, but Rachel does not even know the triage patient has arrived at the unit.

Sometimes it takes an outsider's eyes to see the problems: techs admitting patients, charge nurses being overwhelmed, patients sitting for long periods in a room before receiving nursing care. It is no surprise that later in the afternoon Rachel says in an exasperated tone, "I'm so glad I'm only charge until three o'clock!" She exclaims this just before she leads a "mini-tour" of the unit for a woman and little girl. I write in my notes, "I just think how Rachel is having so much trouble managing everything, and now she's giving a tour!" There are regular tours scheduled for the unit, but nurses are generally not responsible for them. It is not clear who started this tour, but Rachel takes responsibility for it. In other words, the difference in pre-and post-Axiom worlds in the unit is that patients no longer receive the kind of care patient-oriented nurses like Rachel gave them before. There is simply not enough time.

Evelyn

Evelyn has been a nurse for over twenty-five years. For most of her career she has been an OB nurse, with more than half of those years spent at Fuller Hospital. She was the most experienced, patient-oriented nurse I observed. Her patient orientation is likely in part a reflection of her training as a childbirth educator and lactation consultant. She took these roles on for eight years of her nursing career, but the emphasis on education and helping patients clearly stayed with her. She explains that her mother guided her career decision:

> I went with the nursing piece because my mother seemed to think that that's what I would be good at. Because I liked babies she thought pediatrics would be my thing, but then I realized sick babies were not real exciting to me. It was not something that was going to make me happy. . . . So, I decided to go into nursing. I became an OB nurse. That was exciting to me. I really enjoyed being pregnant. I enjoyed all of the information around . . . reproduction and childbearing and raising kids and children, [and] . . . getting those moms and babies off to a good start.

When I asked her about supporting her patients, her answer indicates that she tries to figure out what the patient wants and adjusts her care from there:

> I just kind of try to get a picture of who are these people, and where are their strengths, and where are their weaknesses, and where are their

needs? I don't always get it right, but I try to adjust it and go, and it's a challenge. I've learned that labor and delivery is never the same day twice. . . . You can get the crunchy granola bar natural . . . person to the give me everything you've got, throw it at me—I want every machine, every drug, and I don't want to know. It's a challenge to kind of find the balance for them, to find what makes them feel safe. . . . I mean in the end you want them to have an experience that they're going to remember.

It is also clear from my interview with Evelyn that it's important to her to talk with patients about what they want:

A lot of it has to do with just acknowledging how they feel and trying to get them to verbally give you an understanding. . . . I'll say to them, "So, explain to me so that I understand why you feel this would be important to your care. . . . I have to fill in the gaps, so help me fill in the gaps." Sometimes it's a clear-cut conversation if I say it just like that. Sometimes I have to kind of ask those open-ended questions to get them to give me information that kind of helps me to fill it in, because I don't know how to help them.

Further, Evelyn has empathy for patients, and this is evident from how she ties the way she cares for patients to her own birth experience:

I think I get that advocacy for my patients through the fact that . . . my first experience in the hospital was not what I had expected based on what I learned, who I was, how I was parented. It was my first-ever experience of being a patient. . . . My childbirth classes were in one hospital with a group of childbirth educators and people who kind of taught what I was very comfortable with . . . but I delivered in a different hospital. My experience there was anything but supportive and caring and, you know, it was not a nice experience on many levels. . . . So, I think that I just draw on all of that and try to bring to my families that I care for what I feel is just a positive piece.

This type of reflection is common among patient-oriented nurses: they are empathetic and focus on the experience the patient wants most.

Evelyn, like Rachel, also sees her role as a patient advocate. She tells me about a situation early in her nursing career at a different hospital in which a resident told her to "straight cath" a patient so that he could check the patient's cervical dilation.[13] It is easier to check a patient if her bladder is empty. However, Evelyn refused to do this because the patient was able to walk to the toilet, and therefore there was no reason to catheterize her. She said that the situation escalated to the point that it went to the head of OB, who asked them both to present the issue. According to Evelyn, she told the resident, "Tell him the problem you have with me." The resident told the head of OB that he wanted a straight cath so that he could check the patient's cervical dilation. She said that his complaint immediately dissolved because the head of OB knew that the resident was wrong. Evelyn has a backbone on advocacy issues, which benefits patients.

Evelyn enjoys teaching, and she is good at it. For example, in a January 2014 observation, Evelyn explained charting—postpartum and labor—to me, which takes an inordinate number of keystrokes for the nurses just to get to the right screen. Learning these details makes clear why nurses spend so much time on documentation. According to Evelyn, charting is not intuitive. There is a designation for charting tasks being either active (A) or complete (C). Evelyn demonstrated how anything on the care plan (CP) must be charted, while anything marked as order entry (OE) does not. So, for example, a hepatitis B shot is an OE. That means that nurses do not have to chart it because the documentation of the shot will automatically appear in the patient's record as being ordered and given. Evelyn goes on to illustrate that there is a standard order list that appears when the baby's orders are entered into the system. Evelyn was often followed by orientees, especially once new nurses began to be hired into the unit. No doubt, this is because of her skill and patience as a teacher.

Evelyn Pre-Axiom

During an observation in May 2014, Evelyn was assisting a physician with a circumcision. I observed several circumcisions during my observations, but never did I see such careful care of the newborn during the procedure as I did with Evelyn, which makes sense, because newborn care is patient care. Evelyn explains the FLACC score (face, legs, activity, cry, consolability) to me. The infant receives a score of zero, one, or two on each indicator. The higher the score, the more indication that pain exists. Evelyn explains how this is important, not just for documentation purposes, but also to gauge whether the baby is in pain. She explains that they use sucrose to help the baby with pain. She discusses the patient safety protocol involved with any surgical procedure of writing on the body part involved in the procedure or, if writing is not possible, giving the patient a green-striped ID label that is different from the normal ID label. In either case, the physician checks to make sure he or she has the right patient and is operating on the right body part. This all demonstrates how Evelyn has not only the inclination to help me understand the procedure but the time to do so.

In a second observation of Evelyn in the pre-Axiom period in May 2014, she is caring for a patient being induced at thirty-eight weeks. The patient is pregnant with twins and believes an induction at thirty-eight weeks is healthier for the babies (she has read that the risk of stillbirth goes up for twins after this point), and she hopes to time the birth so that the doctor on call is willing to oversee a vaginal twin delivery (not all physicians in this practice are). Evelyn cares for the patient while orienting a new nurse. Her socialization of the nurse, who has been a NICU nurse before but has no experience as an obstetrical nurse, is remarkable. She tells her at one point, "Don't ask her about discomfort. Say it in a different way, like, 'How are you feeling?' Don't always emphasize pain." She also tells her that with twins the easiest way to monitor the fetal heart rates is to use a scalp electrode to monitor one baby's heart internally and then use external monitoring for the second twin. She tells her this and concludes, "But I'm not a convenience nurse." She monitors both the fetal heartbeats externally and even attempts to connect the patient to a telemetry unit so that the patient can walk while being monitored, but finds that none of the telemetry units has a place to plug in two fetal heart rate monitors. She uses these times to socialize the nurse into her patient-oriented ways. She also cares for the patient in an empathetic way, emphasizing movement, position changes, relaxation, and the use of the birth ball and peanut ball. Evelyn spends much time in the room caring for the patient, feeling her abdomen for contractions, and talking with the patient, her husband, and her doula.

This observation is important, too, because Evelyn is never assigned another patient, not even a triage patient. She has time to take breaks to eat—a late breakfast at around 10:00 and lunch at around 12:30. Thus, although she is busy with the patient and with orienting a new nurse, she is not so busy that she cannot take breaks and have time to eat. The feeling among Evelyn, her orientee, the patient, her partner, and the doula is that of friends, and this feeling is developed over the great amount of time Evelyn and her orientee spend in the room. Having one patient allows for nurses to bond with their patients.

Evelyn Post-Axiom

Times have changed. In a January 2015 observation Evelyn is assigned to a woman who has high blood pressure and signs of preeclampsia, a dangerous condition in pregnancy that, if untreated, may lead to maternal seizures.[14] The unit is busy during both days I observe Evelyn's care of this patient, and Evelyn is fortunate not to be assigned another patient, likely because this patient is being induced for potential preeclampsia, a serious condition. Secretarial staff are stressed, and this stress is at least partially due to only one secretary being on duty during the day (whereas there are usually two). On one occasion Evelyn is in the medication room retrieving Cytotec (an induction agent). A second nurse is also in the medication room. The secretary comes into the medication room—something that rarely happens—and says, "A patient needs help back to bed and another patient needs something, and no one's out there [at the front desk]. I'm all by myself." Evelyn does not respond, but the other nurse tells her, "Well, I have a full assignment on my plate." The secretary leaves the room, clearly exasperated. The NICU staff are stressed as well. On the second day of this observation, a friend of Evelyn's who is a nurse in the NICU tells her that the day before the NICU nurses were strained. The NICU nurse is clearly angry. There had been three cesareans the day before, and one of the cesarean babies screamed all day but no one came to help.[15] She said that the charge nurse, who is responsible for staffing both the LDRP and NICU, did not come to see if they needed help and that none of the NICU nurses even got lunch. Evelyn sympathizes but has no solutions for her.

Evelyn goes to the room to greet her patient. The patient's partner, the father of the baby, is in the room. They are not married, and this is the first baby for them both. Evelyn's care of this patient stands out in her communication, telling the patient everything that she is doing. This is consistent with her philosophy of involving patients in their care and assessing their wishes. For example, early in her care of the patient, Evelyn tells her, "I'm doing the neurological exam because preeclampsia is a neurological disease, and I want a baseline. I need to know after I start this [induction] that things are still the same. Your body is building up toxins." Evelyn also reveals to the patient that she had preeclampsia with her first child and understands what she is going through. For instance, she tells her, "I felt the same way when I had my first baby." She also encourages position changes and shows the patient how to use a peanut ball. Another interesting pattern evident in Evelyn's care of the patient is in how she listens. The monitor is not picking up contractions, but the patient says she is regularly having contractions. Evelyn listens to the patient about this. She palpates the patient's abdomen and confirms that her uterus is contracting. She concludes, "That's why you listen to women, not machines."

Her advocacy also comes through for this patient. On the second day of the induction, the physician orders Cytotec to be placed in the patient's vagina (the medication can be given orally or vaginally). Evelyn carries the pill in her pocket for over two hours, waiting for the midwife to come to the room to place it vaginally. Surprisingly, when the midwife finally arrives, she has a family medicine resident in tow, and the resident places the Cytotec vaginally. It is clear the resident is inexperienced at even checking cervical dilation—she is right-handed and sits to patient's left side, awkwardly reaching her hand across her own body and the patient's body to insert the Cytotec. Evelyn tells me in a hushed voice afterward that residents never place Cytotec because they are not trained to do this and don't have the experience. Later, Evelyn confronts the midwife about this when she finds her in the hall. The midwife admits that she has been pressured by physicians in her practice to let the residents "do more." Evelyn tells her that it is questionable whether the Cytotec was even placed correctly because the patient told her she felt like the exam was different than the others she'd had. Evelyn makes it clear to the midwife that the resident should not place Cytotec again.

The midwife, clearly chastened, deferentially tells Evelyn she will not allow this to happen ever again.

However, Evelyn's advocacy and care for patients cannot save her or them from changes in the hospital. One problem that might seem trivial but has real implications is that Fuller has changed suppliers to save money. One of the supplies to suffer this fate is lubricant, which is used routinely for cervical exams and when a woman is pushing. The new lubricant packets are difficult to open. Physicians have trouble opening them with gloves on and must ask nurses for help. This happens today. The physician tells Evelyn, "I used to do all of this myself, but now it's so hard. It's ridiculously hard. I just can't do it, and I have to have you do it. It's too hard to do." Another time, a nurse used a washcloth for traction to open the lubricant. I witnessed this problem numerous times. Both practices make it more likely that germs will enter the lubricant and possibly cause infection. Further, missing equipment is an ever-present problem, this time for medication pumps, stickers to label IV tubing, a stethoscope, a hammer to check the patient's reflexes, and the paternity information booklet for fathers (the only one available is for mothers and is colored pink).

The most telling observation of Evelyn in the post-Axiom world to indicate organizational changes came in November 2015. Recall the snafu when Rachel was in charge and assigned a triage patient to Evelyn—this is the same day. The triage patient she is assigned (in addition to her post-cesarean recovery patient) is an eighteen-year-old sent to the hospital by her physician because she is term and complaining of diarrhea and cramping. When Evelyn and her orientee, Angela, evaluate the patient, they find that the patient's blood pressure is alarmingly high. Because Angela has been Evelyn's orientee for several shifts, Evelyn turns over more and more responsibility to her. Thus, it is Angela who asks Evelyn if she should "go get a hammer," a request to which Evelyn gives a quick nod. Angela intends to test the patient's reflexes to evaluate whether she has hyperreflexibility, an early symptom of preeclampsia. Angela leaves the room and comes back with a hammer. She checks the patient's reflexes and takes notes. Evelyn asks the patient if she thinks she can pee. She tells her they need a urine sample to see if she has protein in her urine, another sign of preeclampsia. Evelyn puts in a stat lab order. This indicates to the lab that they need to come right away to draw the patient's blood, as there are certain indications of preeclampsia that can be detected in a blood test.[16] It is clear that Evelyn is concerned the patient may be preeclamptic.

While the patient is in the restroom, Evelyn tells Angela, "We need to call the doctor right away to let her know about this, but let's get one more blood pressure and also wait until we dip the urine. Then we'll call." Evelyn tells Angela a trick. She says they can pour the patient's urine over the testing trip (typically the nurse would dip the strip in the urine) in order to keep the rest of the urine uncontaminated so that they can send it to the lab. The strip contains several tests all down the strip vertically. While the patient is in the restroom she also shows Angela how to read the strip. The receptacle, which looks like a small sample paint canister, has the various tests listed in columns along the outside. The tests are timed, and the displayed colors are displayed in such a way that the nurse can turn the canister slowly while holding the urine dip strip vertically against it to compare the strip to the receptacle's colors. The patient returns from the restroom, and Evelyn puts a blood pressure cuff on her and tells her that they are going to set the cuff to take her blood pressure every fifteen minutes.

Evelyn notices that the toco is not picking up the patient's contractions. She adjusts the device as Angela asks the patient if she has any allergies. Then, Evelyn gives the patient paperwork to look over and sign. Evelyn and Angela next turn their attention to the urine specimen. It has been long enough to read the results. Keeping consistent with her teaching role, she holds the strip up vertically and begins to turn the canister slowly and read the results of the various tests to Angela. The findings are normal.

Evelyn and Angela go to the front desk to call the doctor and to finish charting for the cesarean patient they have been caring for since the beginning of Evelyn's shift. The doctor does not answer her phone, and Angela leaves her a message to call her back. They see on the monitor at the front desk that the patient's toco is not working again. They cannot see her contractions. Before heading back to the room to fix it, Angela looks at the blood pressure readings on the computer at the front desk and says, "This doesn't look good." Suddenly, an alarm goes off. A baby's bracelet was taken off for discharge but has not been deactivated. There is a loud argument at the front desk about who was supposed to have deactivated the baby's bracelet. While Evelyn and Angela are still at the front desk, the physician calls back about Evelyn and Angela's patient, and Angela updates her on the patient's status. As they leave the desk, Rachel tells Evelyn that she gave her cesarean patient to someone else so that she can just have the triage patient. Evelyn responds, "I hope someone nice." This is an insightful reminder that, until that moment, Evelyn and Angela were technically still caring for the cesarean patient, something that is hard to do while overseeing the care of a fairly sick triage patient. Persistent high blood pressure in pregnancy is not something to take lightly. Evelyn and Angela go to the patient's room and adjust the toco.

Finally, at almost three o'clock, nearly an hour and a half after Evelyn and Angela abandoned their lunches in the break room, they sit down to eat. However, after taking a few bites of her lunch, Evelyn realizes that the lab has not yet come to draw her patient's blood. She likely would have noticed this earlier had she not been occupied with finishing charting (and teaching the new nurse to chart) for the patient recovering from a cesarean. She gets up and calls the lab on the break room phone. She is clearly frustrated and says into the phone, "If you're shorthanded, you need to let us know because we can draw our own labs. But it just seems to expedite it if someone comes up and takes the blood directly to you." She slams the phone down, clearly angry. This conflict is yet another indication of staff shortages across the hospital.

They finish their lunches in fifteen minutes and return to the patient's room. Evelyn finds that the patient's blood still has not been drawn. She is livid. She continues to chart for several minutes. Seventeen minutes later the lab calls for Evelyn. She tells the person on the phone that she is "putting in notice." This means that she is filing an internal notice that the stat lab was not done correctly. She explains to me that she is doing this to protect herself because she asked for the lab almost an hour ago. Finally, someone from the lab comes to draw the patient's blood.

When Angela spoke to the physician on the phone earlier at the desk, the physician had asked her to put the patient on her left side, an order that Evelyn and Angela turn to implementing. However, there are no extra pillows in the room. Evelyn tells Angela to go to room 12 for more pillows; she thinks that room may have some extras, and it is close to the triage room. Finding extra pillows is a common problem, and nurses sometimes have to search more than one room to find them. Angela is in luck and finds the pillows in room 12. They use the pillows to prop the patient on her left side. While they are doing this, Evelyn continues to wait for the lab results, watching the computer screen for them to appear. They finally do at 4:00, and, thankfully, they are normal. Evelyn and Angela leave and go to the break room and then to the front desk, where they chart.

At 4:20 Evelyn tells Angela to go the patient's room to test the patient's reflexes, but, before she can, a call comes out for a second nurse in room 9, a sign of an imminent delivery, so Evelyn and Angela rush over.[17] Angela wants to see more births, and Evelyn is trying to fulfill this desire, a sign of the responsibility she has orienting a new nurse. But note that this takes them both away from the triage patient.

They come out of room 9 about fifteen minutes later, after the patient delivered, and go back to the triage patient's room. Evelyn sees that the patient's blood pressure readings are still elevated and the blood pressure alarm is ringing again. Evelyn asks the patient, "Are you thinking some thoughts that are exciting or are you nervous?" The patient tells Evelyn that she's nervous. Evelyn asks, "Are you nervous about the birth, about the baby?" The patient answers, "Yeah. I'm nervous and excited." Evelyn tells her, "Well, you're just normal!" What is not being said is that because Evelyn and Angela interrupted a trip to the triage patient's room by going to the delivery, the triage patient was without nursing care for some time. It is likely the beeping alarm had been going off for much of that time, which may have contributed to the patient's anxiety.

The father of the baby asks if the patient can eat, but Evelyn says they need to talk to the doctor first. She is supposed to be in at five o'clock, which is fifteen minutes away. Evelyn and Angela continue to document and take the patient's vital signs. The physician does not show up until 5:30. By then Evelyn has filed paperwork to admit the patient, and Evelyn and Angela have moved the patient from the triage room to an LDRP room. It is clear that her blood pressure is consistently high and that the physician will induce her labor tonight.

An analysis of this observation demonstrates that it is symbolic of change at the hospital. Evelyn is tasked with caring for two patients for almost her entire shift, and both are high need—one recovering from a cesarean and the other a patient who is potentially preeclamptic. As a result, Evelyn barely has time to eat lunch. After trying, and failing, to care for both, Evelyn is finally relieved of her cesarean recovery patient. She only has the triage patient to care for, but the patient is "sick" in the world of antenatal care because of her persistent high blood pressure. Short staffing also affects Evelyn because she cannot get a quick lab drawn. In fact, she had to file notice (i.e., a formal complaint) because the stat lab was drawn too late, something that was due to the lab being short staffed, likely a result of cutbacks. In other words, these cutbacks affect patient care. Evelyn had to spend her time calling about the lab and, if the results had been ominous, this could have had a drastic impact on the patient. Further, she has the responsibility of orienting a new nurse. These conditions do not allow Evelyn to buffer patients from changes at the hospital, although, no doubt, she tries.

Lori

Lori is a nurse who almost escapes categorization. She advocates for patients but otherwise provides care in a lackadaisical way. This includes her lack of focus on documentation and charting. That means that she is clearly *not* a process-oriented nurse because paperwork is something she only does grudgingly. Other nurses complain that she used to be a good nurse but has given up; I cannot confirm that assessment because I only watched her work over a three-year period, and she had been at the hospital for over ten years. Nonetheless, she advocates for patients readily, shielding them from what she views as inappropriate care, which leads me to place her in the patient-oriented category.

In a November 2015 interview Lori explains that she always knew she wanted to be a "maternity" nurse, and being pregnant with her first child confirmed that interest. She says, "So I just went from one class to two classes to three classes and did all my prerequisites for nursing. At that point, I think I knew I wanted to be a nurse. . . . With my pregnancy with [my first child], I just loved it, the whole thing, and . . . I was always interested in woman's health anyway." She went to nursing school and worked as a nurse at two different hospitals, one of them in the postpartum unit, before coming to the OB unit at Fuller Hospital more than ten years ago.

However, the conversation quickly turned to how much she hates her job with the recent changes in the hospital. In her own words she has given up, having just turned down a job at another hospital. She decided that she just could not give up her seniority, and she had been given a co-hort schedule that gave her large chunks of time away from the hospital, a condition she says was necessary for her to stay. Yet she is still the most consistent and vocal advocate for patients who do not want interventions or who have been subjected to what Lori considers unnecessary proce-dures. In that way she is a stalwart. It matters not whether the patient she views as being railroaded is assigned to her or someone else. If she thinks the patient is being pressured to have a procedure that the patient does not want and/or that Lori views as unnecessary, she speaks up.

Numerous examples illustrate her advocacy. She tells me that she once had a resident tell her he was going to check the cervical dilation of a patient. She followed him to the room and did not let him perform the check because she believed residents do not have the skill to check a patient's cervical dilation.[18] She mentions another form of advocacy one day when she overhears a nursing-student supervisor talking to students about the need to ensure a baby is breech (*not* presenting in a vertex or head-down position) before performing a cesarean for breech presenta-tion. Lori interjects into the conversation that she always does an ultra-sound before a woman has a cesarean for a breech baby because she has seen too many cesareans for a breech baby when the baby isn't breech. One of the students asks how she makes sure the ultrasound is done. Lori tells her that she puts the ultrasound unit in the operating room. They all laugh, but there is no doubt that Lori is serious.

One day, Lori ends her shift with the care of a triage patient, whom she has to retrieve from the emergency room. Although ER staff mem-bers will transport patients to any other unit of the hospital, they will not transport a patient to the OB unit out of fear that the woman might give birth on the way. She makes the long walk to the ER, and the pa-tient walks with her back to the unit. She takes the patient to a triage room to admit her as an observation patient. She is kind to the patient in ways that show empathy. For example, when she asks the patient if she has picked out a pediatrician, the patient says that they go to a walk-in clinic. Lori tells her:

> Well, you know, the benefit of picking a pediatrician is that you'll have
> consistency of care and, so, if you have a well visit or your baby's sick,

you'll have someone to call. The other good thing about going to a pediatrician's office versus a walk-in clinic is that the people tend to be less sick. They often have separate waiting rooms or waiting room areas for kids who are sick versus kids who are there for well visits. So, you might . . . just think about it.

Even in collecting information from a triage patient, Lori advocates and educates when she sees that a patient needs this from her.

Lori Pre-Axiom

Several examples in the pre-Axiom period demonstrate Lori's activism and also her time to advocate. In an October 2013 observation, there is a patient scheduled for an external cephalic version, a procedure in which a physician, guided by ultrasound, attempts to maneuver a fetus not presenting in a vertex or head-down position into such a position by applying external pressure. Lori is assigned to this patient, and the procedure is successful. Lori tells the physician she will monitor the patient for 60 minutes. The physician tells her that the patient must stay in the unit for four hours. Lori responds by telling the physician that the protocol is only sixty minutes of monitoring. The doctor tells Lori that she is going to treat the patient like someone who has fallen down—a four-hour observation. Lori asks if the patient has to be monitored (meaning a fetal heart monitor and contraction monitor will be used continuously). The doctor says no. Lori replies, "Why keep her four hours if you're not going to monitor her? She could abrupt either way."[19] Lori does not win this dispute, but she does attempt to pressure the physician to let the patient go early. She also makes clear to everyone who witnessed this interaction at the front desk that the physician is being irrational.

Another example comes from a January 2014 observation. A patient who had given birth and been home afterward for only a few days was sent back to the hospital by her physician when it was found in an office visit that her blood pressure was quite high. The physician on call for the practice mentions a few times in conversations at the front desk that she wants to "straight cath" the patient, which leads nurses to collectively raise their eyebrows because they see no reason for a catheter.[20] The patient is mobile and, even with an IV pole, can go to the toilet by dragging the pole behind her. Even with the incredulousness all the nurses clearly displayed, Lori is the only nurse to question the physician, not only raising her eyebrows but also asking "Now, why would you do that? Why do you need to do that for magnesium?" The doctor relents.

A final example of Lori's advocacy is very patient focused. This comes from a February 2014 observation. The focus is on a patient who had given birth the day before and had lost quite a bit of blood. Her physician recommends a blood transfusion. However, once the patient reads the risks of the transfusion, she decides against a transfusion. Nurses and the patient's physician alike are frustrated. They think she needs a transfusion and are disturbed by her "waffling" on the decision. Lori is the only nurse to stick up for the patient. She says, "Well, you know, if you need a transplant, if you've had a transfusion, you would have lots of antibodies in your body [which might make the transplant more likely to fail]." This is a striking example of her advocacy.

Yet, I saw, too, what the other nurses reported about Lori's taking shortcuts to many tasks on the unit and often avoiding doing work, trying instead to find others to do the work for her. One example involves the practice of nurses requesting my help. For example, Rachel once asked me to go to the supply room to get a pink basin for a patient who was vomiting. She knew she might need another basin, and she was busy dealing with the patient and disposing of the vomit. In this case, asking for my help enabled her to provide better care to the patient. Yet Lori often asked for help with tasks she could and likely should have done herself. For example, one day I am standing at the front desk. Someone from IT had come to fix a computer in room 3. Lori turns and asks me, "Who's in room 3." I tell her I don't know, but it also struck me that she was sitting at the desk and a push of a button would bring up a screen with the information she needed. Another time, Lori parks a scale by Julie. Lori's patient had just delivered, and Lori knew that Julie's patient was close to delivery. Julie will soon need a scale. Lori says to Julie, "You can have this [the scale] if you'll clean it." Other nurses would have cleaned the scale before delivering it to another nurse, especially a nurse who was just about to start pushing with the patient, a time-intensive activity. Another example happens one day when a resident comes to the desk and says to Lori, "We need backup for mec." It is important to recognize that residents are very poorly integrated on the unit, so the resident likely had not been given instructions on how to deal with requests such as finding "backup for mec." This request refers to finding NICU nurses and/or physicians to go to the room. No doubt, Lori could have done this more easily than could the resident because she knew exactly whom to find, but she offers no help to the resident other than to tell him, "Go to the NICU." In other words, Lori has not totally given up. She still advocates for patients, often when no other nurse is willing to do so, but she takes noticeable shortcuts that lead to her less-than-stellar reputation. Yet, an analysis of the situation suggests that before Axiom pulled out of the acquisition attempt Lori had time to advocate and to care for patients. She took shortcuts, no doubt, but they were not dictated by the hospital's situation itself, but rather her own personal preferences.

Lori Post-Axiom

I followed Lori on back-to-back days in November 2015, both busy days that are good examples of how the unit has changed. Before her shift even starts on the first day, she tells me she is moving to the back desk because the front desk is "just too chaotic." As Lori departs for the back desk, another nurse, Julie, tells me, "I took two days off last week to get out of this madness!" These observations set the tone in this new era. Not only are there more patients, but there are new nurses, residents, and nursing students. Chaos is a constant description of what the unit is like now.

Lori is assigned a patient in preterm labor who is being induced. The patient is at thirty-four weeks gestation, her water has broken, and her baby is not growing well (intrauterine growth restriction or IUGR). The first-time parents are nervous, and Lori attempts to put them at ease. To set the mood of her interactions with the patient, when Lori goes to the room to introduce herself, the fetal heart rate monitor is beeping because it has run out of paper, and Lori imitates the beep in a song as she changes the paper and stops the beeping. She tells the patient that the physician is in another patient room, but she will find her and come back with a plan for the day. Before she leaves, she asks the patient if she would like the lights turned off and offers to cover the monitor screen, both offers the patient accepts. When Lori finally finds the doctor she asks, "Can I walk her?" The doctor says yes, and Lori goes to find a telemetry unit, which will allow the patient to walk while Lori continues to monitor the fetal heart rate and the patient's contractions. She is advocating for this patient. The patient has not asked to walk, but Lori knows that walking will help dilate the patient's cervix. The patient's water is broken, and the clock is ticking on how long the physician will give the patient to dilate before suggesting a cesarean.

Lori finds a telemetry unit and takes it to the patient's room, a practice nurses often follow to ensure they have a working telemetry unit when their patient wants to walk. Lori asks the patient if she would like to walk. The patient seems uncertain, but Lori encourages her. She says, "Well, think about it at some point. It will really do you good to get your contractions going. It's hard to get them going when you're lying down." She leaves to let the patient consider her offer. When she goes back thirty minutes later, the patient is sleeping. Thirty minutes after that, she is successful at getting the patient to walk. Her care and encouragement of the patient continues through the rest of her shift.

Lori is assigned to the same patient the next day. The patient has dilated to five centimeters but has developed a fever, not uncommon for someone whose water has been broken for over twenty-four hours. The parents exhibit quite a bit of anxiety, which Lori deals with well. For example, when Lori comes to the room to change the Pitocin bag, which has run out, she says, "Bells and whistles!" The father of the baby tells her that the bag is empty. She tells him, "Don't worry. I have it covered. I have a new bag right here." She talks in a calm way and ignores that the father seems not to trust that she is taking care of the patient. She exhibits confidence that sets the tone for a calm day.

Although the patient has a fever, because she is dilating the physician tells her they will attempt a vaginal birth. Beyond the fever, the fetal heart rate is decelerating at times, and Lori is constantly using position changes to "fix" the strip. These position changes are difficult because the patient has an epidural and, thus, cannot easily change positions. Lori uses her body strength to help the patient change positions. The patient's cervix reaches eight centimeters of dilation. Shortly later, Lori suspects that the patient is fully dilated (ten centimeters). Lori decides not to check the patient's dilation because, she says, "If I check her now and she's fully [dilated], then we have to start pushing, but the baby may not be down low enough. And she might have to push too long, and they might get anxious, especially with the variables [in the baby's heart rate]." Thus, she is helping the patient by allowing her contractions to bring the baby farther down the birth canal, and, during this process, she continues to help the patient change positions. She is allowing the patient to "labor down."

After thirty minutes of the patient's "laboring down," the physician checks the patient and determines that she is ready to push. Lori ensures that the patient's legs are supported, NICU has been called, and a gas-powered neonatal resuscitator known as a neopuff is in the room. The baby is only at thirty-four weeks gestation and is expected to be smaller than an average baby at that pre-term age. They also suspect that the baby may have trouble breathing. The baby is born in eighteen short minutes and, after being intubated, is transported to the NICU. Lori stays and cleans the room while the physician waits for the patient to deliver the placenta. She compliments the patient on her slender abdomen: "I think you can wear pants. It's just not fair!" She finishes cleaning the patient, cleaning the room, and taking the trash and dirty laundry down the hall.

After everything is clear, Lori goes to the back desk and begins to chart for the patient. While she charts, she talks to me about the hospital and how it has changed. She says that she used to love the hospital, especially compared to the two others she worked at before, and that she was so happy with her job. But she doesn't feel that way anymore. Instead, she tells me that she hates her job. She explains that there is not enough staff support on the unit and that there is an expectation that nurses will care for more patients. For example, she tells me that there are more active labor patients with the addition of the new practices and that sometimes the charge nurse even has deliveries. She also discusses the problem of not having enough rooms, and she ties this problem to staffing as well. Although 3 West has six rooms, the charge nurse has to look at the staffing for the next shift. If there aren't enough nurses to staff the unit in the current *and* in the upcoming shift, they cannot open it. Further, high-level administrators have told the nurses that they may not open 3 West unless there are only two open rooms left in the unit, and this includes triage rooms. In fact, perhaps Lori's insight was foreshadowing, because this exact situation unfolds later in the day. The charge nurse says, "We have two rooms plus one triage room, but we can't open 3 West because we only have three [nurses] on tonight and no call. And we have an induction tonight at five o'clock." Lori suggests that she might want to cancel the induction. The charge nurse says, "It's not my problem. I'm off at three o'clock," a clear way of passing on the problem. They do not open the 3 West unit.

The changing organizational environment also affects Lori's care of the patient. The scanner that electronically documents patient medication fails to work properly for her. This causes her anxiety because she has been "talked to" because of her low (78 percent) compliance rate—the goal for compliance is above 90 percent. When she cannot get the medication to scan and overrides the system, she goes to tell the OB clinical coordinator as a way of protecting herself from further attention to her low compliance rate. The OB clinical coordinator tells Lori to call IT. "I'm buried," she tells Lori. The nurse manager had taken a required furlough day, and the coordinator had to do both her own job and the nurse manager's job. Lori continued to have problems with the scanner throughout her shift and was sure to talk to the clinical coordinator each time, which meant taking time away from her patient and from required documentation. To make matters words, Lori finds that the ampicillin she needs to give the patient had not been mixed by the pharmacy, so she has to mix it herself. She mixes it, but when she starts the patient safety protocol, she finds that the pharmacy has not verified the drug. This means that Lori cannot scan it and again has to override the system. The clinical coordinator to whom she once again talks tells her that she should have had another nurse verify the medication for her rather than overriding the system. As we walk away from the clinical coordinator, Lori tells me that this is a new rule she has never heard before. Lori is affected by staff shortages in other units in the hospital, in this case the pharmacy. Nurse shortage is also an issue. Lori needs another nurse to assist her in getting her patient out of bed following the birth. She can't find anyone to help. She goes to the back desk, the front desk, the break room, and the back desk again. She finds no nurses and sighs. Finally, she finds a nurse just coming onto the night shift and asks her to help with the patient. She agrees.

Lori finishes her documentation, but she works on it sporadically rather than methodically. For example, although she is to take the patient's temperature every two hours because the patient's water is ruptured, she is not careful about the timing of this. Her experience as a nurse leaves her less worried about temperatures because she knows other signs of fever to look for, like elevated heart rate.[21] After the shift, she asks me to look through my notes so she that can update her documentation with such things as what time she turned the patient and checked vital signs.

Further, Lori deliberately avoids having a resident follow her or orienting a new nurse. This is consistent with what I have documented as the nurses' frustration with the organizational change at the hospital in terms of nurses training doctors and new nurses. A resident comes up to Lori when she is at the back desk and asks if he can watch her patient. It is clear he is hoping to see a birth. She tells him, "I have a patient who . . . I don't know that she's really wanting males in the room, and then I have a sociologist." I thank her for not deserting me. She says, "You were here first." Later, she avoids orienting a new nurse, claiming that she had a resident follow her the day before. Another nurse softly challenges her, saying "She [pointing to me] followed you yesterday, not a resident." But Lori does not back down. In other words, Lori finds ways to avoid the extra labor of orienting nurses and teaching residents.

Throughout the day, there is talk about the employee pension and 401(k) plans not being funded. Nurses discuss this constantly, and it is clear they are not happy. As though trying to keep nurses from thinking about the financial constraints directly affecting them, administrators have devised a ploy called Munchy Monday. Two administrators bring a big basket of candy to the unit and offer the doctors, nurses, and support staff treats. The nurses are polite but clearly not won over by such a tactic, feeling it is a pathetic reward for good unit outcomes. The day after Munch Monday, Lori tells me, "You know those two people who came yesterday—they were so fake—with candy and telling us what a good job we were doing. Just so fake." In fact, right after the administrators left with their basket of candy the day before, the nurses started talking about cuts to benefits and pension—they were not distracted by Munchy Monday. When we're at the back desk, Lori tells me that there were nurse layoffs in the OR, and that there was a rumor that two nurses from OB would be laid off, "but we nixed that and it never happened."

Lori is frustrated by her increasingly hectic and demoralizing work environment. She tells a break room full of nurses that she used to recommend to women that they give birth at Fuller Hospital, something she can no longer say with any sense of honesty. Her frustration is clear, and she links it to upper-level changes at the hospital that affect her work life and care of patients.

Wendy

Wendy is a high-profile nurse because of the way she presents herself. She is loud and opinionated but in a manner that makes obvious she cares about her patients. She has an infectious laugh, and her voice can be heard from the far side of the unit. If anyone needs to find her, they only need listen. Wendy is a nurse who aspires to move up from her current position. She has an associate's degree and is just a few hours shy of a bachelor's degree. She plans to finish her bachelor's degree and then complete a master's degree to become an advanced practice registered nurse (APRN). She remembers from her childhood always having the desire to be a nurse, which was cemented when she received training in high school as a certified nurse assistant. However, obstetrics was never her focus. Rather, her first love was pediatrics:

> I was challenged greatly by my [pediatrics] clinical instructor at the bedside in regard to med doses for children, which can be pretty tough calculating. And, so . . . I knew that I was good at it, and the families really received me well—dealing with families who have sick children is not easy because the parents are distressed and they cannot do anything to fix it, and they're relying on you to make their child better. So, well, I felt like I found my place—and [the local children's hospital] was under fire at that time, and they had a hiring freeze.

She described how she came to an open house at Fuller Hospital and was recruited by the OB nurse manager, who offered her a job in the OB unit. She accepted and had been at the hospital for several years at the time of the interview.

When I asked her about supporting her patients, she mentioned the importance of getting to know them:

> To me, it's you have to get to know the patient and their family. You have to get to know what their hopes and dreams are, what they're willing to do on their end to help foster that birth that they want, working with me, working with the provider. . . . It's getting to know them first, and then, yes, it's definitely altering as we go along. So, you have to adapt, and there's a lot of changes that happen very quickly. . . . When it doesn't happen, it's all about emotionally being there for them at the time they need you the most, because things didn't go according to the plan that they wanted.

A common virtue of patient-oriented nurses is their ability to perceive and to be attentive to the diversity of patient desires, wishes, and characteristics. Notice, too, how Wendy talks about emotionally supporting patients.[22]

Wendy sticks with this philosophy when socializing other nurses. For example, fetal death is hard to deal with, and it takes an emotional toll on nurses who support patients following such an unfortunate event. When another nurse is assigned a patient whose fetus died in utero, Wendy helps the nurse see how she can care for the patient, even though the nurse says that she is not the kind of nurse to cry with and hug patients. Wendy tells her, "You know, as nurses, we're supposed to be stoic, and we're not supposed to show emotion. So, it's, you know, it's okay to go in there and be empathetic but not cry. You don't have to cry with her. You just have to show that you understand what she's feeling."

Wendy Pre-Axiom

In a March 2014 observation, Wendy is caring for an obese patient being induced for a "big" baby. The baby is predicted to be seven pounds, twelve ounces. Inducing a woman for a baby this size is not consistent with professional guidelines, and the nurses are very frustrated with the situation.[23] The patient does not want an epidural—she had given birth to two babies already without the use of regional pain medication and did not intend to use it with this birth.

Wendy spends most of her time with this patient. Due to the patient's size (maternal habitus is how Wendy refers to the patient's weight characteristic), the fetal monitor does not consistently pick up the fetus's heart rate. Because the patient is being induced with Pitocin, according to hospital protocol she must have continuous fetal monitoring. This protocol is due to the potential of Pitocin to lead to fetal distress if contractions are too strong, as I discussed in the prior chapter. Wendy instructs the nursing student who follows her for the first half of her shift that it is important to continuously trace the fetal heart rate if the patient has Pitocin. She says, "They will tear you apart if your documentation isn't done right," referring to her supervisors. Wendy stays in the room so that she, or more commonly the nursing student, can adjust the monitor every few minutes.

It is clear that Wendy knows comforting ways to help the patient through labor. For example, when the patient has a contraction, Wendy tells her to "melt like butter." When she has trouble placing an IV in the patient's arm, she calls the lab and asks for a phlebotomist to place the IV. She tells the patient she is doing this because she doesn't want to "make you a pin cushion." Taking this step—which requires the nurse to wait for the phlebotomist to arrive—is an indication of Wendy's patient orientation.

Another indication of her orientation is that she gives information to the patient that other nurses often don't. She tells her that the phone in the room does not ring after 8:00 p.m. for the privacy of the patients. She advices the patient that, if her partner does not have a cell phone, he should take the number of the direct line into the room so that he can call her if he leaves. She tells them that discharge is at 11:00 a.m., but that when it actually occurs depends on how busy the unit is. She continues by telling the partner that there is a cafeteria but to watch the hours so that he does not go when it is closed. She also tells them of a nearby car-seat check, performed by a local police department to ensure car seats are appropriately installed in vehicles, done every Wednesday morning. In the middle of this information exchange, the patient has a contraction. Wendy seamlessly goes from giving the patient information to telling her to breathe and blow the breath away. She then tells her, "I saw your tense face. Your face was all tense. I'm going to take a picture of it if you don't stop doing that." She laughs, an indication that her admonishment is all in good humor. The patient's partner says he'll post the photo on Facebook and Instagram. Wendy tells him, "No, no, no! Just show it to her!" She is undoubtedly a patient advocate.

Having time to devote to this patient also gives Wendy time to suggest position changes, even going to get the coveted peanut ball, which she commandeers early on because she knows there are several labor patients on the unit and she wants to make sure her patient has access to the ball. She indicates that this is especially important since the patient does not have an epidural and movement can help alleviate labor pain. Wendy also encourages the patient to get up and walk around several times, but the patient always declines, insisting that she is more comfortable in bed. Wendy's encouragement of walking stands in contrast to process-oriented nurses who prefer their patients to stay in bed so that it easier to monitor the fetal heart rate and the woman's contractions. Wendy takes the patient's refusal in stride, making a homemade "hot pack"—a steaming hot towel sandwiched between two dry towels, all put into a large ziplock bag—to ease the patient's pain.

Wendy is good at relating to patients and finding topics to discuss with them, in this case, hair. The patient is African American and has beautiful, intricate braids in her hair. The nurse asks who does her hair. The patient answers, "I do." The nurse, who is white but has a biracial daughter, tells of her struggles to pull her daughter's hair back, attempting a connection with the patient by telling her, "My daughter is half black." They continue to talk about hair, all while Wendy and the nursing student attempt to keep the fetal heart rate documented continuously. At the end of the conversation Wendy announces, "Someone is going to come and break your water so we can put an internal monitor in. That way we don't have to torture you." It is questionable who is being tortured. The patient seems to be enjoying the conversation, but Wendy has gotten quite behind on documentation because of her time in the room. Documentation needs to be completed before the end of her shift. She tells me throughout the day that she is behind on documentation and will have to reconstruct what happened throughout the day. She is uncomfortable with this, but not so much that she takes time away from her patient to work on required documentation. That is a key dividing characteristic between nurses I call "patient oriented" and nurses I call "process oriented."

When I observed Wendy, missing supplies had reached a critical level, something that happened even in the pre-Axiom period. She is missing a pair of scissors for the delivery. I have discussed this issue with nurses and doctors and have come to understand that there are usually two sets of scissors in the instrument kit used for a birth, one straight set and one curved set.[24] Usually the straight scissors are used for cutting an episiotomy and umbilical cord and the curved set is used for cutting sutures. When Wendy prepares the hospital bed for delivery by removing its end, she remembers that she has only one pair of scissors. She had mentioned to the nursing student earlier in the day that they were short a pair of scissors and needed to get an extra pair, but they never did. The charge nurse comes into the room. When Wendy tells her she only has one set of scissors, the charge nurse tells her, "I got by with one pair yesterday," indicating that missing a pair of scissors is not an isolated problem. The delivery kit is sterilized as one unit. Thus, it is difficult to find an extra pair of scissors, and this puts the patient at risk of infection. In this case, the patient pushes only three times before the baby is born. She requires a few sutures for a tear in her perineum. The physician uses the same pair of scissors to cut the baby's umbilical cord and to cut the sutures. And, this is not the only item that is missing in this birth. The unit is out of medication commonly given to a woman after birth to ease the pain and swelling of her perineum. Wendy discusses this with another nurse, who tells her that the father of the baby should go to a pharmacy to get Preparation H or Tucks for the patient. Wendy is frustrated because, of course, she should be able to provide medication for the patient from hospital supplies.

Wendy Post-Axiom

Wendy's behavior after organizational changes demonstrates the effect of such shifts on nurses. In a January 2015 observation, after the Axiom deal disappears, the unit is madly busy, and the nurses fret about the impending March 1 date when two new practices will start deliveries. There are four labor patients and a scheduled cesarean, and the unit is chaotic. Wendy gives up an "easy" mother-baby pair for a woman who had been her labor patient three years ago. Wendy explains, "I kind of treat them like family." Taking care of one mother-baby pair with few complications is much less time intensive than caring for a labor patient, which shows how Wendy puts patient care first. This decision also affects Wendy negatively because the nurse who took the mother-baby pair is called into a scheduled cesarean, and Wendy is assigned to care for *both* the labor patient and the mother-baby pair. The mother-baby pair received very little attention throughout the day, partly because the labor patient is not easy to care for—the fetal heart rate has variable decelerations and, when the physician breaks the patient's amniotic sac, the amniotic fluid has meconium mixed in. Meconium is the baby's first bowel movement; if it makes its way to the baby's lungs (fetuses "breath" amniotic fluid in utero), it may block the baby's airways. A NICU nurse will be present at the delivery to suction the baby's lungs immediately after delivery. Also, the patient is "high anxiety" and asks repeatedly throughout her labor if everything is okay, if the baby is okay, and if she's doing everything right.

Wendy spends her day going to the patient's room to turn her to help with the fetal heart rate decelerations. She intermingles trips into her pair's room when vital signs are required or when the baby's blood sugar needs to be checked (a new policy means that Wendy has to check the baby's blood sugar more frequently than she used to). Because of all this, Wendy's documentation falls behind. At one point during the day she says, "I haven't even had a chance to chart on my strip," which is basic documentation that nurses are to stay current on when caring for a labor patient. She also is forced to deal with the always-present problem of missing equipment. In this case, she needs to stock an aspirator on the baby crash cart (in the room because of the baby's potential for meconium aspiration) and cannot find the right size aspirator in the supply room. She wants a size 4.0 and has to settle for a size 3.5. There is good news in that the unit did buy a few new spotlights, and this room has one of them. The physician, who is middle-aged, jokes that the light will be here until he retires, showing that physicians share the notion that supplies and equipment are always in short supply and rarely replaced. The labor patient is in a room with a dripping sink that Wendy hopes will be fixed after the birth, when she will have time to call engineering. Until then, there is a constant drip, drip, drip in the background.

What goes on during this day is that everyone is busy, not just Wendy. No nurses get to take a lunch break. Jennifer is charge nurse. She sits down at the front desk with a container of soup, looks at me, and says, "This is the closest to a lunch break I am going to get today." Jennifer has to document for the unit's records that no nurse takes a lunch break because all nurses are now required to clock out for a thirty-minute lunch break, a relatively new policy. In fact, in a January 2014 interview Julie told me that if nurses are too busy for a lunch break they will be paid and that they are not required to take a lunch break She also told me that eating lunch standing up or watching a monitor does not count as a lunch break. It has to be a true break from patient care. In other words, the new policy requiring nurses to clock out for a thirty-minute lunch break is a significant change in policy.

Wendy stays past her shift to care for the labor patient until she gives birth. She is not paid for this time but rather clocks out at 3:30 and stays to help, uncompensated. Wendy explains that she used to be able to stay clocked in for a delivery, but that the administration has "cracked down on this." She calls her children's father to pick them up from the bus stop so that she can stay. She provides care, like giving the patient a cold cloth and encouraging her. She also advocates for the patient. When at 3:45 the physician asks when the patient started pushing, Wendy answers, "Well, at 2:30, but she didn't really have feeling, and we just dropped the epidural. So, she's just having feeling now. It hasn't been over an hour. We really shouldn't count that first bit of pushing because she couldn't feel." She is buying the patient time, similar to how Amy did, highlighted earlier in this chapter. She puts a rolled towel behind the patient's back to help turn the patient on her side when the fetal heart rate drops. The baby is born quickly and cries right away. The concern with aspiration is gone when the baby cries. It is too late at this point to suction the meconium out of the baby's lungs since she has already inhaled and shown that she can breathe with an enthusiastic cry. Wendy gushes when the baby is born and stays for another thirty minutes, helping the nurse who took over her nursing tasks. The nurse who took over says, "You know, we should have a policy for two nurses for every delivery," indicating how she benefited from Wendy's help. Note that Wendy stays and helps even though she has had a busy day and has childcare responsibilities of her own. She put her own personal life on hold for this patient. This is an indication of what patient-oriented nurses do for their patients. Wendy is not even being compensated for her time.

Times have changed at the hospital, and nurses like Wendy are filling in the gaps by trying to give patients the care they deserve. Wendy did not get a lunch break, struggled to find the right equipment (finally settling on an aspirator that was the wrong size), and stayed with a patient for delivery without compensation for her time. Yet, notice that even though Wendy protected the labor patient, the postpartum patient received little care because Wendy did not have time. Once times became tight, nurses are pulled in too many directions at once to provide optimal care.

Lillian

Lillian is a wonderful and empathetic nurse. She emphasizes patient care over hospital rules, although I do not mean to suggest she does not follow the rules. She just bends them a bit here and there and documents when she has time rather than on the "hospital's schedule." Lillian came to nursing as a second career:

> I became unhappy for a number of reasons with [my first] career and decided that I would go back to nursing school. . . . When it came time for my clinical rotation in school, . . . I was just amazed at how miraculous birth was . . . and I was just sold. Fortunately, when I got out of school the nursing market was wide open. . . . I knew that I wanted to do OB, and I was pretty sure that I would choose to do it at the hospital that I work at now . . . if I could have it my way, and, fortunately, they had an opening.

Nursing was a second or backup occupation for a number of the nurses. The occupation offers flexible scheduling and allows the expression of nurturing skills, something for which women are socially rewarded. It was also common for nurses to have a family member who had been a nurse and, thus, the job seemed natural for them. Many nurses, both process and patient oriented, explained how they had fallen in love with OB.

Lillian cares for patients in a way that sets them at ease. She uses humor and sometimes even silliness to help patients deal with IV placement, blood draws, and cervical dilation checks. She has favorite songs she sings to them, unannounced, and she also makes up raps about her job at the hospital. Patients typically crack up at her performances.

When I ask her about advocacy, she gives me specific examples of how she advocates for patients. For instance, she tells me of a time when she arrived at her day shift and was assigned a patient who was receiving more than the maximum dose of Pitocin specified by protocol. She tells me that there was a new nurse caring for the patient who had increased the Pitocin even though the patient was only four centimeters dilated and "wasn't doing much." Lillian turned the Pitocin off for an hour and let the patient rest. She then turned the Pitocin back on. The patient dilated and had a vaginal birth. Lillian believes this outcome was due to her turning the patient's Pitocin off. She ends the story by saying "It's my job to be an advocate." She follows with another example. She tells me, "There is one doctor who likes to do episiotomies. We do things really carefully. We time when we call that doctor in. We don't call the doctor in until the baby's head is practically out." She tells me that, one time, the doctor had scissors in her hands and Lillian said to the patient, "Oh, look at your perineum! It's stretching so much. I don't think you're going to need an episiotomy." The doctor put the scissors down. "There are doctors we really have to guard the patients from," she concludes. Lillian wants to be involved in a profession that benefits society, and she sees her care of patients as doing just that. She even goes so far as allowing a nurse orientee to practice giving IVs on her, which I found absolutely amazing, especially because the orientee was clearly nervous and caused Lillian significant discomfort, perhaps even pain, in the lesson.

Lillian Pre-Axiom

I start here with an observation from March 2014. Lillian is caring for a patient who had delivered the previous day and is struggling with breast-feeding and a triage patient who is being evaluated for bleeding and low fluid. Lillian also has a student following her during the care of the women who had given birth, and this complicates her schedule because, beyond caring for the patient, she is expected also to teach the student.

An interesting anecdote illustrates the busyness of the unit before and after Axiom withdrew the acquisition offer. In this pre-Axiom observation, Lillian is also working per diem (i.e., she picks up shifts rather than being a regular employee) in another hospital on the postpartum unit. She does not like it and talks continually throughout her shift on the subject. She explains that she does not like her per diem job because she always has four mother-baby pairs. She is assigned a tech who does some of the care for her—taking vital signs, helping the patient out of bed, making sure the birth certificate application is signed—things she does at Fuller Hospital. She says that it is not that she likes doing mundane tasks, but that doing these things allows her time to bond with the patient. This discussion is a bit foreboding because once the new practices start delivering patients at Fuller in March 2015 (one year after this observation), nurses are routinely caring for three or four pairs with *no* help from a tech, more than replicating the conditions Lillian despises at the other hospital.

Lillian focuses on her postpartum patient in ways that are typical of the nurses I term patient oriented. She tells me before she walks into a patient's room that she always makes sure the patient is not asleep, and she follows through with this dictate by tiptoeing into the room and backing out when she realizes the patient is asleep. As Lillian walks back toward the front desk, she hears a ruckus, followed by the charge nurse exclaiming "What the fuck!" The patient-safety protocol that requires nurses to scan the patient's ID, their own ID, and the medication is not working in any of the rooms. None of the computers in the patient rooms will scan the medication. Instead, the nurses are told by an IT employee that they will need to wheel in what the nurses term "a cow" (a portable computer). This new patient-safety protocol was unveiled in the unit the day before, and it is not working. Nurses have to use the portable computer or override the system. Overriding the system may seem easy enough, except that the system keeps track of overrides, and administrators discuss overrides with nurses whose percentage of overrides is "high," as I mentioned earlier in the chapter when I highlighted how this happened to Lori. The IT problem is not solved quickly. At least one IT employee is on the unit the entire day trying to fix the system. When I ask Lillian about the new system, she tells me, "I can't describe how much I don't care about this. It is to make the documentation idiot proof." She goes on to tell me that nurses are very careful and make sure the medication they are giving patients is done correctly. She says that this is just adding another time-consuming step for nurses.

I follow Lillian into the patient's room. The patient is awake this time. Lillian asks the nursing student if she is okay to take the baby's temperature, and the student says yes. But, then, Lillian has another problem. She had earlier pulled a rolling cart into the room. The cart has an attached thermometer and a basket in the front, which usually holds a portable thermometer. Lillian prefers the portable thermometer because it is easier to use on babies. The attached thermometer has to be reset depending on whether it is being used on the mother or baby, and resetting it takes several steps and much time. Lillian tells the student to use the portable thermometer to take the baby's temperature but then realizes it is not in the basket. "Oh, did someone steal it?" she exclaims. She realizes later in the day that none of the carts have portable thermometers; they have been "taken away." I was in the hospital the day before when a representative from the company selling the attached thermometers was in the unit. It was clear to me that the hospital is transitioning to only using the thermometers attached to the cart. This information neither found its way to all the nurses nor, consistent with the majority of changes occurring, were the nurses consulted about it. Lillian expressed her frustration with this situation several times during her shift. She tells the student later, after they leave the room, "I never use these [attached thermometers]. They're so hard to use. It's so much easier to use the other ones." The secretary overhears Lillian and says, "Yeah, yesterday they came and took them all, and we're not getting them back."

Regardless, Lillian takes care of the patient throughout her shift, with a focus on helping her breastfeed. This is the patient's second child, and she did not breastfeed her first. She expresses an interest in breastfeeding but tells Lillian that she supplemented the baby last night with formula because she is concerned that the baby latches too long and is not getting enough milk. Lillian is patient and quells her fears. She explains that the baby is getting colostrum, not milk, and that many babies cluster feed, which causes milk production since nipple stimulation causes a woman's body to produce milk. She explains this repeatedly and, when the baby spits up, Lillian points out its yellow color to the patient, telling her enthusiastically, "That's the color of colostrum!" She also gives the patient tips, like that it is easier to breastfeed a baby at night than it is to mix together a bottle of formula.

When she is in the hall later in the day and a call comes from the patient that she wants a bottle, Lillian rushes to the room and asks her about this request. The patient tells Lillian that the baby is continuously sucking. When Lillian asks if her nipples are sore, the patient admits that they are. Lillian says, "What about a pacifier? I don't know why I didn't think of this before!" She brings a pacifier to the room, and the baby readily takes it. Lillian tells the patient, "I'll take the heat from [the lactation consultant] for the pacifier." Lactation consultants typically dissuade breastfeeding women from using artificial nipples because they believe that artificial nipples may cause the baby to have breastfeeding problems, although empirical research does not support this fear.[25] Lillian, however, talks to the lactation consultant about why she gave the baby a pacifier and how it will facilitate breastfeeding. She does this outside the room, saving the patient from having to hear any frustration from the lactation consultant.

Lillian soon turns over the postpartum patient to the nursing student and her supervisor, which seemed odd to me. Nonetheless it happened. She had a triage patient who was sent to the hospital for low fluids after seeing her physician for bleeding. She is at thirty-four weeks, and Lillian is to figure out whether she is in preterm labor. The patient speaks limited English, and her partner interprets for her. However, this does not go well, and they seem not to be able to agree on whether the patient had been in the hospital a few days earlier. Lillian tells me in the hall that the patient is frustrating, sometimes taking several minutes to answer a question and other times telling her information she doesn't need. Lillian has to deal with this situation in a way that supports the patient, and she does. However, her frustration with the hospital is apparent when she finds that the kitchen is out of apple juice, which the patient had requested, and she later cannot find a thermometer to use. She finally finds a thermometer, substitutes cranberry juice for apple juice, and delivers the patient her beverage.

The midwife checks the patient for cervical dilation and finds that her cervix is thick and closed, indicating that she is not in preterm labor. The midwife decides to discharge the patient. The patient requests Tylenol for a headache before she is discharged. Lillian goes to get Tylenol but finds that the midwife has not entered the order. She uses a trick to deal with this. She tells me that she's going to get the Tylenol and then put the order for it in the computer because if she puts the order in first, she'll have to wait a few minutes for the pharmacy to approve it before it will be dispensed, thereby delaying the medication. Lillian gets the Tylenol and gives it to the patient with some water. She then goes through discharge papers with her.

Notice that in this time Lillian is caring for a mother-baby pair for nearly her entire shift. When she is assigned a triage patient, she is immediately relieved of her pair. She can focus on one patient at a time. This is almost unheard of after Axiom withdraws its acquisition offer.

Lillian Post-Axiom

In the post-Axiom world of Fuller Hospital, Lillian is still the caring and patient-oriented nurse she was at the start of my observations, but she is distracted. The distraction comes from the basic uncertainty that entered her work life when Axiom pulled out of the acquisition deal in December 2014. She has a patient who is very quiet, and Lillian provides care in a way typical of her orientation—offering a birth ball (even demonstrating its use), suggesting position changes, and commandeering a working telemetry unit so the patient can walk while being monitored. She has quirky practices that, on the one hand, seem silly, but, on the other hand, set patients at ease and cause a laugh. For example, the patient she is caring for broke her amniotic sac at home and is still dripping amniotic fluid. When Lillian goes to her room to introduce herself at shift change, she finds a trail of amniotic fluid on the floor. As she wipes it up, she talks to the patient, telling her that she is wiping up her "baby bunny trail." This is silly but makes the patient laugh, putting her at ease. A few minutes later, the patient gets out of bed to use the restroom. Lillian removes the fetal heart and uterine contraction monitoring belts so that the patient can walk to the bathroom. While doing this she says, "Be free, be free," making swaying motions with her hands.

However, in private conversation with me and in her discussions with other nurses, the uncertainty of the hospital takes precedent. She talks about two concerns, and other nurses chime in to support her. The first is that the Axiom acquisition fell through, and now they do not know what will happen next. The second is that nurses know that two new practices are joining the hospital in March—just two months away—and Lillian and the other nurses expresses angst over how the unit will change as a result.

Lillian is the first to say something to me about the new practices. She tells me less than an hour after I arrive on the unit that a practice with doctors and midwives in a nearby town is going to start deliveries at Fuller Hospital in March 2015, as will a practice of two midwives. The rumor is that the obstetric/midwife practice is moving its deliveries to Fuller because the hospital in the nearby town banned VBACs. However, some of the nurses also have a suspicion that the timing of the practice coming to the hospital has to do with the hospital's financial situation needing to be bolstered. I share their suspicion. I had spoken to a midwife a few years ago who was with this practice, and even at that time she told me how, with the hospital having been recently acquired, the acquiring hospital system had shut down their VBAC deliveries. I am suspicious about the timing, too, given that the VBAC ban at the hospital had been in place for at least two years. Why would the practice move their deliveries to Fuller Hospital at this particular time? A likely explanation is that they were wooed. Two hundred new deliveries every year is a significant revenue boost to Fuller Hospital.

Lillian quickly follows by telling me about how the Axiom deal falling through has affected her life: "What's happened since Axiom withdrew their offer to acquire the hospital is that our salaries have been frozen and they no longer match our 401(k) contributions." She says this in an exasperated, hushed tone. She then says that just as they are experiencing these financial consequences for their own lives, they found out that a $3,000 signing bonus has been offered to a nurse employed by another hospital if she accepts a night position in the unit. The nurses found out about the bonus because one of the Fuller nurses is friends with this nurse and referred her for the job. The idea of a new nurse getting a signing bonus while nurses already employed at Fuller Hospital are facing a salary freeze is a huge point of contention. I heard about this over and over, and I empathized with the nurses' frustration.[26]

This conversation continues as we walk into the break room, where Lillian tells me that her continuing education courses are no longer going to be reimbursed. She wants to take a class to keep up her obstetrics certification. She explains that nurses have always been able to take one class per year and have the class reimbursed by the hospital. She was planning to take a class, but when she inquired about reimbursement she was told that it would not happen. She is frustrated because in order to maintain her certification in obstetrics she needs to attend continuing education classes. The courses also help her to stay up-to-date on the latest research in obstetrics. She is reflective, wondering whether the $198 price tag was the reason she had been refused.

She continues her discussion about Axiom pulling out. She says, "It is really, really bad that [Axiom] stepped back because they were going to infuse cash into the hospital." I asked her why, given these circumstances, the hospital is hiring nurses. She indicates that the hospital was supposed to have a two-year emergency plan to fall back on if the Axiom deal did not go through, and that part of this was bringing the new group to the hospital. I wrote in my notes, "There was talk throughout the day from the nurses and at a crew meeting about where they were going to put these extra two hundred deliveries; how they're going to deal with them; how they're to staff them. And the nurses are not too excited about the new nurses coming on, saying they didn't care for the idea because they would have to precept the new nurses." In short, I find a markedly different environment for nurses, and Axiom's pullout is the cause of the change.

During this observation a crew meeting is held in which the nurse manager, who is not typically at these meetings, tells the nurses that Axiom is going to come back to talk with the governor, because Axiom has been pressured to do this—the implication is that Fuller Hospital executives were the ones applying the pressure. However, she says that the board has met and sent out a letter of intent to other interested partners, including organizations that had already shown an interest in acquiring Fuller Hospital. The organizations were given ten days to respond. She also indicates that hiring is underway, especially for the night shift, and that the hope is that renovations to the unit will be underway soon. When questioned, she confirms the rumor of a $3,000 signing bonus being given to a nurse who accepted a night-shift position. Later in the day, the nurse who brought up the bonus issue at the crew meeting tells me that the nurse manager called her into her office and admonished her for "bringing staff morale down" by discussing the bonus. The signing bonus is an indication of the administrators' knowledge that the night shift may become problematic, even unsafe, due to more patients and low staffing. In this economically struggling hospital, offering a signing bonus should be seen as an indication of crisis.

Lillian leaves the meeting and immediately goes to find an IV pump for her patient. She says, "Let's rob that from room 7 or 11. We need more stuff because we have to borrow it all the time. It's like robbing Peter to pay Paul." She finds a pump, "steals" it from the room, and takes it to her patient's room. She needs the pump to start the patient on Pitocin, something the patient's doctor has ordered to augment her contractions. Lillian makes sure to get the patient out of bed to go to the restroom before she starts Pitocin. She also encourages the patient in a gentle and encouraging way to walk around and use telemetry. She tells the patient how beautiful the baby looks, referring to the baby's heart rate, and follows by saying, "This is my favorite room." The patient asks if all the rooms aren't the same. Lillian answers, "Well, no, this is a corner room, and it's a bit quieter. Invariably, I always have nice births in here." Lillian finds a good telemetry unit and hides it in the crib because, she explains, only two telemetry units work.

I spend the rest of Lillian's shift with her, following her as she cares for this patient, explaining how to use telemetry ("This is your little pocketbook"), how to drag along the IV pole as the patient walks ("You look stunning, gorgeous!"), and how to navigate the room ("You have to pop a wheelie to get over this hump into the bathroom"). Her care is always about the patient. But she is distracted by the changes going on in the hospital, which other nurses commiserate about in conversation. Focusing on these changes takes her time away from the patient, even though her care is still exemplary.

My last observation of Lillian is in November 2015. I cannot express how busy the unit is and how busy Lillian stays. My notes are a whirlwind of what Lillian did, and reading them now only confirms how busy the unit was compared to earlier observations. The new practices are taking a toll on the nurses and the unit. Lillian is caring for a patient being induced for a medical indication; she is on fourth day of induction and frustrated.[27] Besides the usual struggles of being induced early when one's body is not ready, this patient struggles with anxiety over cervical exams and IV placement. The patient is assigned to Lillian, the perfect nurse for such a patient. I describe how she makes the patient's day much easier.

To start, Lillian decides not to call the physician overseeing the patient's care until the patient eats breakfast. She tells me that the physician will tell her not to let the patient eat, so she wants to make sure the patient eats before the call. When the patient's tray is slow to arrive, she calls the cafeteria to expedite its arrival. When I ask her about this, she tells me that the patient needs energy before she starts Pitocin. She does not agree with the hospital policy that laboring patients may not eat and may only drink clear fluids, but says it will never change because it is set by the anesthesiologists who will always remember the one patient who ate during labor and aspirated during a cesarean. She works around this policy, as she has done today. Another way she works around it is to tell patients in early labor that hospital policy is that they cannot eat but that if they were to eat some crackers or a granola bar when she is out of the room, she would never know about it. This is a kind of "wink wink, nudge nudge" way of encouraging patients to break a policy and eat.

The patient has a nonreactive fetal heart strip. This means that the fetal heart rate is in the normal range but flat, with no accelerations. The fetus could simply be asleep, but a consistently flat strip can indicate fetal distress.[28] Protocol is such that a nurse may not start Pitocin on a patient until the strip is reactive. This patient's labor has been plagued by a nonreactive fetal heart rate, and nurses have tried various tricks to make it reactive. Lillian turns the patient from side to side, jiggles the patient's uterus, and talks loudly, hoping to wake the fetus. She does all this while assuring the patient and her husband that everything is fine. The husband asks a number of times if everything okay, and Lillian assures him that it is and that she is just waiting to see the baby's heart rate accelerate.

When he seems overly anxious, she tries distraction, by talking about trees outside that have something white wrapped around the bottom of their trunks, by asking about the nursery colors, by playing a name game—what would your name be if you were the opposite gender and your first name started with the same letter as your first name? For example, we decided that my name (Theresa) would be Thomas. She is a genius at distraction, and Lilian's use of distraction and humor is a deliberate choice to help patients.

She realizes that she has to change the patient's IV because it is puffy, something she is hesitant to do because the patient has already had three IVs and has significant anxiety about the procedure. She starts the placement and, as she prepares to place the IV needle, Lillian breaks into song, surprising the patient. Then, when she "blows a vein" (goes through the wall of the vein), something she says she hardly ever does, she immediately goes to find another nurse to give the patient an IV. A more common practice is for the nurse to try again. However, Lillian, realizing the patient's anxiety, decides to find another nurse to help relieve her anxiety.

She continues this type of care of the patient throughout the day and helps the patient stay encouraged by saying things like "Let's get this birthday party started!" She "steals" equipment from another room, for example, an IV pole with a push handle that the patient requests to make walking with the IV pole easier. She subtlety critiques Ashley, the nurse who told the patient the day before that IV penicillin burns and gave the patient three separate IVs. Lillian is able to stop the burn of the penicillin with extra IV fluid and is frustrated that the patient had been told to expect a burning feeling. She is also critical of the patient's having so many IVs, especially because IV placement gives the patient anxiety. This is a demonstration of the ways process- and patient-oriented nurses differ in how they care for patients.

It's no wonder why the patient's husband asks more than once whether Lillian can stay with them until the baby is born, and he is only partially joking. At one point he asks Lillian pointedly, "Can you stay with us?" She jokes that she has been on shift since 3:00 a.m. (she had been called in to work a 3:00–7:00 a.m. call shift) and is nearly spent. However, what he seems to mean is could she stay in the room instead of leaving at that particular moment. Lillian likely knew this but joked because she cannot stay. She has been assigned a triage patient who is headed to the OR for an emergency cesarean. Although she cannot stay continuously with the patient, she does stay beyond her shift by over twenty minutes so that she can sing to the patient while the physician checks her cervical dilation.

This is just one way Lillian deals with consequences of the hospital's financial straits. She has to go to another room to find Pitocin stickers, which allows her to label the tubes that deliver Pitocin to the patient, an important safety practice. Later in the day she has to steal a pump from another room when her Pitocin pump won't stop beeping. She also is pulled in different directions, being assigned not only a high-maintenance labor patient but also a triage patient who ends up with an emergency cesarean. She eats at the front desk—technically a banned practice—because she does not have time to sit in the back room to eat.

A frustrating indication, to the nurses, of financial distress and the hospital administration's trying to rally the forces, so to speak, is when, during every shift on a day I am following Lillian, two administrators roll a cart into the unit, on which sits a treasure chest. Nurses are given keys to the treasure chest if they can give the administrators any of the Perinatal Care measures (used by the Joint Commission, an organization that accredits and certifies U.S. hospitals—although they didn't say that). The measures are:

- PC-01: Elective Delivery
- PC-02: Cesarean Section
- PC-03: Antenatal Steroids
- PC-04: Health Care–Associated Bloodstream Infections in Newborns
- PC-05: Exclusive Breast Milk Feeding
- PC-05a: Exclusive Breast Milk Feeding Considering Mother's Choice

Only a few of the keys unlocked the treasure chest, which is filled with five-dollar gift cards to various retailers (e.g., Dunkin' Donuts, Panera Bread, Starbucks). Nurses who give a correct answer and do not have a key that opens the chest are allowed to pick a snack bag of chips. They play along, but, as soon as the administrators leave, the nurses express derision: their pay is frozen and yet the hospital finds the money to buy gift cards and snack-sized bags of chips? How does this silly game make up for the increased strain on their work and financial lives?

Lillian's work life has changed. She must juggle patients and, even though patients adore her, she cannot give them her uncommitted time. Further, being taxed with ever increasing patient loads is not the only problem. The uncertainty of change also distracts Lillian and the other nurses. They spend time talking and discussing the changes in a way that pulls them from patient care.

Conclusion

Patient-oriented nurses are empathetic to patients and feel the stress of trying to absorb changes at the hospital in order to shield their patients from their effects. However, as much as they try, shielding patients is not always possible when things out of their control happen, like short staffing. Kerry, a patient-oriented nurse, in a December 2015 interview told me of a night where she was pulled in two directions: "There was a night over the summer where I had a patient who was naturally laboring. She was like, four to five, and then I had a patient with an epidural who was nine centimeters . . . and they were short-staffed. I was like, is that a mistake? And they're [like], 'Nope.' . . . I'm like, 'Okay, but I'm delivering the nine-centimeter one,' like, 'What are we going to do with the one in the tub?'"

A consequence of the ACA is pressure on hospitals, especially small, non-profit hospitals, which were put under increased financial duress when the ACA was passed. With new performance measures that are tied to reimbursements, these hospitals have a hard time staying above water, particularly when, at the same time, they are financially stressed by changes in state policies. Organizational theory predicts that managers will respond to these changes. Yet, what my analysis shows is that the response does not benefit the nurses or patients. Patient-oriented nurses feel the change in ways that do not allow them to deliver patient care in the way they would like. They attempt to buffer their patients, but there is only so much one nurse can do.

4

Process-Oriented Nurses

> The hardest part of working with patients sometimes is the birth plans. . . .
> Some things can be unacceptable, ridiculous. People aren't in health care,
> [and they] want this, want that. . . . It's like this is not the way it works
> 'cause we have to do things for safety, something that's on our license.
> (Jennifer)

All nurses contribute to patient care, whether they are patient or process
oriented. Each type of nurse fulfills different organizational needs, and
the nurses tend to balance each other out. Process-oriented nurses, like
Jennifer quoted above, are concerned when patients break hospital protocols, which sometimes happens with birth plans. The focus of these
nurses is on strictly following and enforcing hospital protocols and rules
and documenting that they have done so. This is what they view as their
most important role in caring for patients.

I want to make clear at the beginning of this chapter that it is not
my intent to demean nurses I term process oriented or to suggest that
they are less valuable to the hospital than are patient-oriented nurses. In
fact, with increasing profit pressures and demands to document every
element of a patient's care in the hospital, process-oriented nurses are
increasingly important to the hospital's organizational goals. It may appear that I negatively evaluate nurses *because* I show how they spend less
time with patients and less time engaged in nurturing behavior. In the
context of labor and birth, women giving birth are expected to embody
gendered norms of caring behavior.[1] There is no doubt that nurses are
also subject to such normative expectations. Yet, if we step away from
these gendered expectations, one will see throughout the chapter that
process-oriented and patient-oriented nurses balance each other in
terms of meeting organizational objectives and goals.

One gets a sense of the complementary values in both types of nursing from an example involving Heather, a process-oriented nurse, and

Lori, a patient-oriented nurse I highlighted in chapter 3. Heather is the charge nurse on a busy day, one characterized by room pressures and a nurse shortage (two nurses had called in sick). As charge nurse, Heather must think ahead about rooms and whether she will need to reassign nurses who are already assigned to patients in order to staff an emergency cesarean. That is part of the job of the charge nurse. There is a patient laboring with twins. Her water is broken, which increases risk of infection, but otherwise her labor is going well. Heather is watching for any complications that might lead to a cesarean. A cesarean is more likely with multiples, and Heather is worried about staffing for a potential surgery. The nurses are looking at the monitors, and Heather announces that the twins' baseline heart rate is elevated. This could be a sign of infection. I write in my notes, "Heather clearly wants to call a cesarean, perhaps to resolve the uncertainty of not knowing how this birth will end up." The following is a conversation that takes place between Lori and Heather following Heather's announcement of the twins' elevated baseline heart rate:

> LORI: Has she had a prior c-section?
> HEATHER: This is her first birth.
> LORI: So, no. Baseline change?
> HEATHER: She has a one hundred temp.
> LORI: Get an oral read. I don't trust ear thermometers. If she's going to become infected, it will be evident.

Lori, in the language of nursing, is telling Heather that a slightly elevated fetal heart rate baseline and a low-grade fever measured with an ear thermometer are not reliable indicators of infection. Her question about whether the patient has had a previous cesarean is important. This would be the patient's first or primary cesarean. In the United States, fewer than 3 percent of women with a previous cesarean go on to give birth vaginally in a subsequent pregnancy.[2] Lori is reminding Heather about this dire statistic with her question. She is also protecting the patient from an early cesarean, which would likely be the result of an official declaration that the patient's uterus is infected. Lori tells Heather that if the patient is infected this will become evident over time. In other words, she is keeping Heather from encouraging the physician to decide on a cesarean too early. Lori helps Heather to see how waiting is consistent with protocol, thereby balancing their views.

Three hours after this interaction, the patient has a cesarean. The twins are fine, and Lori's advocacy allowed the woman to continue her labor for three additional hours, a likely benefit to her and the baby. For example, there is evidence that labor before a primary (or first) cesarean makes a future vaginal birth more likely.[3] Lori advocated for the patient. Heather strictly followed protocol. Both fulfilled hospital goals, just different ones. This chapter focuses on process-oriented nurses, who internalize the organizational goals of documentation and expedience.

Something also to note about process-oriented nurses is that they are keenly aware of liability risk. All nurses are trained in liability management and know that following protocol is key to preventing malpractice claims. However, this risk seems to be more real to process-oriented nurses, who tend to integrate this concern into their daily behavior. This chapter focuses on how process-oriented nurses were affected by the same rapid organizational changes as were patient-oriented nurses. It should be clear throughout the chapter how process-oriented nurses are deeply affected because changes in the hospital make malpractice claims more likely as basic patient safety standards are not always met. Because these nurses have a strong concern over this issue, their work lives are thrown into upheaval as a result.

Jennifer

Jennifer is the epitome of a process-oriented nurse. When I interviewed Jennifer in November 2015, she had been a nurse for nearly twenty years. For the first two of those years she was a nurse on a med-surg unit. She told me that for those two years she was just biding her time, waiting for a position in labor and delivery to open. Yet Jennifer did not have an early desire to be a nurse. She came to nursing through her own experience giving birth to her first child.

> I wasn't really bent on working full-time when I got out of high school or going to college. So, I just . . . kind of [took] . . . entry-level jobs, you know. I worked as a cashier, a cashier supervisor. . . . But then I started to realize—I'm going to have to work my whole life. I need something

that pays well, and I want to do something that I can use my intelligence for. . . . I had my daughter when I was [in my early twenties], and I loved my labor nurse. She helped me so much . . . and I remember thinking "I think I could do that job. I would like to do that."

Developing an interest in being an OB nurse based on one's own experience giving birth is not uncommon. Note the similarity Jennifer shares with Evelyn (highlighted in chapter 3), who became a nurse because she was *not* supported in the way she would have liked during her own first labor and birth.

Jennifer earned an associate's degree, going part-time for six years. She tells me how frustrated she was by how long it took her to earn her diploma:

I had no choice, and I remember . . . feeling discouraged and saying "Oh, it's going to take so long, and it will probably take me six years." And my grandmother said, "Those six years are going to go by whether you do this or not." . . . And then I found out later, after I was a nurse, my grandmother told me that she had always wanted to be a nurse, and when she graduated high school, she walked down to the hospital and said, "Hi! I'd like to apply for a job to be a nurse." And she had no idea that you had to go to college. And there was no way that her family could afford to do that, so she never did. . . . Little did I know, I was kind of living the dream for both of us.

In other words, Jennifer's entrance into the field also held a personal meaning.

An interesting aspect of Jennifer's orientation is how often she emphasizes bad outcomes that patients have had, often tying them to overreaching birth plans. This is one indication of her being a process-oriented nurse—the patient's plan interferes with common protocols and practices, and this bothers her. She shares an example of a birth plan gone wrong:

This hospital kind of advertises itself as a birth center, where basically I would equate it to the way people plan a wedding. They have something in their mind, it's going to go this way, and they don't want to veer off their plans that they've spent nine months making. So, [when] they come in the door, they have a plan. I don't want monitoring. I don't want any vag[inal] exams. Some of them say, "Don't say the word contraction. Do not offer me pain medication." And, you know, we did have that situation where this couple, the woman was forty-two weeks pregnant. It was IVF [in vitro fertilization]. She was over forty years old—already high risk—and didn't want to be induced. . . . Finally, she agreed to this induction, but she kept taking the monitor off, and the baby didn't look good all night long. Long story short, she was refusing a c-section. Finally, after they couldn't find a [fetal] heartbeat—and I don't know how they convinced her to finally go for a c-section—it was too late. And the baby ultimately died.

Jennifer presents a cautionary tale, but, of course, fetal death is rare for any woman, including women with birth plans. Yet, I found it common of process-oriented nurses to focus on birth plans as problematic, perhaps because some birth plans ask nurses to break protocol. In Jennifer's understanding of caring for patients, hospital rules reign supreme.

The process-oriented perspective is consistent with much training that nurses receive on how to prevent liability risk, and Jennifer's orientation also protects the hospital from liability. Jennifer fully embraces hospital rules as necessary for the safety of patients. Because she has internalized the rules as part of her role, hospital administrators do not have to worry about enforcement of the rules. Jennifer keeps to the rules without the need for such supervision.[4] Another excerpt from our interview demonstrates this relationship when Jennifer says, "Sometimes in the other OB group . . . they're like . . . 'Okay, we'll let you get away with this and let you get away with that,' and . . . that kind of steps on our toes, too. You're caught between a rock and hard place between doing your job and doing what the patient wants."

Jennifer Pre-Axiom

I observed Jennifer on my second day of observational research at the hospital in June 2013 when I was still new to everyone. She is not enthusiastic with my request to follow her, but Julie, the charge nurse on this day, vouches for me, saying to Jennifer, "She won't bite!" Jennifer agrees that I can shadow her while she cares for a patient on the second day of an induction. She is supportive of patients, but just in a different way than patient-oriented nurses are.

The patient is being induced for Rh disease. Blood Rh factor is inherited and makes one's blood "positive" or "negative." The concern comes with women who are Rh negative and who become pregnant by a man who is Rh positive. In such a situation, the baby may be either Rh positive or negative. If the baby is Rh positive and the fetus's blood comes in contact with the mother's Rh-negative blood (during pregnancy, labor, or birth), her blood may develop antibodies against the Rh factor, a condition called Rh sensitivity or Rh disease.[5] In future pregnancies these antibodies may destroy fetal red blood cells. Although Rh sensitivity can be prevented in future pregnancies if the woman receives a shot of Rh immunoglobulin (i.e., RhoGAM) during pregnancy and shortly after birth, not all women receive this medication. Infants whose mothers have Rh sensitivity must be monitored closely after birth to prevent hemolytic anemia, which, in severe cases, can lead to neonatal death.

Jennifer explains to me how serious this disease is for the patient and, especially, for the baby. Yet the patient and her husband seem in good spirits and do not ask questions about what will happen after the birth and how the baby's health will be ensured. Though this seems strange to me, Jennifer explains that the patient and her partner likely do not understand the severity of the disease. She confesses that she did not understand the disease well until she read about it in preparation for this patient. This is the first patient she has cared for in her many years of nursing who has had it—a sign of the prevalence of RhoGAM in preventing Rh sensitivity.

It is the physician's role to discuss such a topic with the patient, and I am sure that the couple was informed in prenatal care about the disease. Although a patient-oriented nurse likely would have either indicated to the physician the patient's lack of understanding, encouraged the patient to ask questions, or, herself, would have explained more to the patient about the condition, Jennifer is a process-oriented nurse. She is making sure to monitor the patient appropriately and document her care of the patient. This is her goal. This example distinguishes process-oriented nurses from patient-oriented nurses.

Another example of Jennifer's process orientation is that, although the patient is being induced and indicates that she wants to walk around,

Jennifer does not work to make it happen. The patient is being induced with Pitocin, and it is an established protocol that a woman receiving Pitocin must have continuous fetal heart rate monitoring.[6] The OB unit at the time had three telemetry units—one new unit and two older, less reliable, units—which allow patients to move around and nurses to monitor the fetal heart rate remotely.[7] Patient-oriented nurses typically make sure the new telemetry unit is waiting in the room for a patient who wants to walk so that it will be available. The nurse from the previous shift had done this for the patient, so the new telemetry unit is already in the room. However, when another nurse asks Jennifer if she can use the new telemetry unit, Jennifer gives it away easily, walking into the patient's room and indicating to the patient that she needs to "borrow it." She later retrieves one of the old units but finds, not unexpectedly, that it does not work well. She does not spend time tracking down the working unit and negotiating with the other nurse a sharing arrangement if the other patient is using it, something that nurses often do. Rather, she complains throughout her shift about how the telemetry unit's not working affects her ability to monitor the patient reliably. Her focus on monitoring patients is typical of process-oriented nurses, who view strictly following protocol as essential. Telemetry makes this task much more difficult, which explains why Jennifer does not make it a priority to monitor the patient using this method.

Jennifer explains to me how her frustration with the situation is tied to liability concerns. She says, "This is my license," and "It's the law; she's on Pitocin." She's here referring to hospital protocol as "the law." If the patient does not have continuous monitoring and there is a bad outcome, Jennifer may be faulted for not following protocol, which would leave her vulnerable to blame in a malpractice civil lawsuit. Jennifer tells the patient and her husband that they "must have" continuous monitoring. After leaving the patient's room, however, she refers to the machine as the bane of her existence and laments to a patient-oriented nurse who complains that her patient will not walk, "You're lucky. Mine won't get in bed." Process-oriented nurses prioritize documentation and following protocol over the wishes of patients when granting the latter makes following protocol difficult.

Jennifer spends much of her time socializing with other nurses and doing personal tasks, such as scheduling a medical appointment for a child, looking at photos on her Gmail account, and looking up and demonstrating various exercise moves. The socializing aspect of Jennifer's work life is also evident in another situation. She is asked to pick up a shift, but, before she agrees, she looks to see who else is working during the shift. She only wants to pick up the extra shift if her friends are working during the same shift. She views a perk of the job as getting to spend time socially with her friends, other nurses, while on duty. Although patient-oriented nurses also socialize at work, especially in the pre-Axiom period, it is not to the extent that process-oriented nurses do because patient-oriented nurses spend less time at the desk and in the break room and more time in patients' rooms.

What should be clear, however, from these examples is that much of Jennifer's behavior is consistent with the administrative goals of the hospital. She is careful to make sure she can document the fetal heartbeat continuously, suggesting that if the reading becomes too difficult to pick up she will "harass" the patient. She is joking, but Jennifer understands that when Pitocin is used during labor, malpractice suits may result if there is a bad outcome and the use of Pitocin will likely be linked to the bad outcome. A Google search for "Pitocin and malpractice" produces dozens of links, and the research literature also suggests that malpractice suits involving an allegation of the misuse of Pitocin are typically successful.[8] Thus, Jennifer's focus on monitoring is consistent with the hospital's administrative goal of preventing costly malpractice suits. Another way that Jennifer furthers administrative goals is by *not* insisting that her patient walk. The dated telemetry units are not an issue for Jennifer because she does not focus on the mobility of patients. These units are expensive and, thus, Jennifer's lack of focus on mobility means she is not pushing the hospital to buy expensive equipment. Further, her emphasis on social relations to other nurses serves as a distancing mechanism from patients, justifying and reinforcing her role as enforcer of administrative protocols, the essence of her process orientation.

Jennifer Post-Axiom

I observed Jennifer in January 2015. As an indication of how different things are, Jennifer tells me, "It's like we got different jobs . . . without ever having left." On this day, a night nurse I had not observed but who had heard about my research talked to me for a few minutes at shift change. She tells me, somewhat prophetically, "It's good you're here. You will likely see lots of changes going on."

The talk of the unit is about pay freezes and the change to the hospital that will come on March 1. In fact, "Wait until March 1" is a nurse mantra, commonly uttered as they look ahead to changes they know will likely make their jobs more difficult. This is said in such a way that, for example, if the floor is busy, a nurse says something like, "You think this is busy? Wait until March 1." News has recently trickled down through the administrative mechanisms of the hospital that the Axiom deal has fallen through. The nurses for the most part favored the acquisition because they believed there would be an influx of capital allowing hospital administrators to update and purchase needed equipment. They blamed the governor for the deal falling through, saying that he had insisted on onerous conditions that left Axiom little choice but to pull out. It is interesting that one of the conditions would have protected hospital employees from layoffs, a benefit to nurses.

Jennifer and another nurse talk at the beginning of the day in the break room—a common place for camaraderie because it is more private than the front desk—about the pay freezes. They discuss how their salaries are frozen at the same time that the "big wigs got big bonuses." They ask why they should bear the brunt of economic pressures at the hospital and why the executives should not share in the pain. Jennifer tells of a story in the newspaper that detailed how the CEO of DHN had gone to the state's governor to ask for economic assistance but that the governor had said no because the CEO and some other "higher-ups" in DHN had taken bonuses. "That's good!" Jennifer exclaims. Although I have not been able to identify the article to which Jennifer refers, there is evidence that the governor was not sympathetic to cries for help from hospitals because of the "bloated salaries" of their executives.[9] This anecdote demonstrates the animosity of the nurses toward the hospital administrators, which is a common view among the nurses.

Another nurse, Lauren, tells similarly of how she took offense at the senior administrators' being paid bonuses when the bonuses nurses have always received—for picking up unexpected shifts and coming in quickly when requested—had recently disappeared. Short call was a bonus that nurses received for arriving at the unit within forty-five minutes of a request.

Lauren explains, "If my boss called me and said, '[Lauren], can you come in and help?' . . . If she called at 1:00 [and] I was here by 1:45, we got short call, which was an extra two hours of pay. So, if I stayed for four hours . . . I got paid for six hours." She explains that a short-notice bonus also recently ended. Short notice is defined as a nurse's being given less than twenty-four hours' notice of when she needs to cover a shift. If this happened, the nurse was paid an extra dollar per hour. Lauren tells me, "Then all of the sudden, both of those—short notice and short call—were gone. We could not punch in for them anymore. So those two tiny incentives . . . were just gone. Gone."

Another issue that came up in this observation of Jennifer is how anesthesiologists feel the pinch of change, too, which, in a snowball effect, causes more pressure on the OB unit. Jennifer talks with an anesthesiologist who is leaving the next week for a better position at another hospital. They discuss how the OB unit at Fuller Hospital is going to be particularly "squeezed" in March once the new practice starts. After the anesthesiologist walks away, I ask Jennifer if she knows why the anesthesiologist is unhappy and leaving her position at Fuller. She explains that the anesthesiologists are not employed by the hospital but rather by an anesthesiology practice that is based in another town, and that the practice "works them like dogs." She says that two other anesthesiologists had recently given notice that they were leaving. Their departure has direct implications on the OB nurses because the unit does not have a dedicated anesthesiologist. Nurses have to call the OR when a woman wants an epidural. Jennifer tells me that if all the anesthesiologists are working on another "case" in the OR, women must wait quite a while for an epidural. She mentions that this reflects negatively on their patient satisfaction evaluations, something the hospital is increasingly concerned with, given the ACA mandates that link Medicare funding to such evaluations.

Soon after this discussion about the anesthesiologists, a triage patient arrives. The patient's physician had called the unit to let them know that the patient is potentially in preterm labor at thirty-two weeks. Her physician sent her to the hospital for the nurses to "rule out labor." Jennifer has to hunt down the prenatal record because the secretary is out for the day. The patient has "white-coat anxiety." I ask Jennifer what that means, and she tells me that the patient is anxious around doctors and that, because of this, her blood pressure might be high in health-care settings. We go into the triage room, and the woman is visibly nervous.

The patient wants to be reassured that everything is fine and to go home. She cringes when Jennifer, in the course of regular patient assessment, takes her blood pressure. It is easy to see how her anxiety may cause high blood pressure. Jennifer puts the cuff on the patient's arm and sets the machine to take her blood pressure, but the cuff does not inflate. The patient asks hopefully, "Is this a new kind of cuff? They usually squeeze my arm, and I can feel my pulse. I don't like it." Jennifer says, "Well, it might have a hole in it." She is visibly frustrated, telling me that first the toco (the contraction monitor) had not been restocked—we had to go looking for one—and now the blood pressure cuff is not working. This is a theme throughout my observations: missing and broken equipment and supplies are a constant source of frustration for the nurses. She leaves to find another blood pressure cuff and comes back with one she took from another room. The patient is fine and not in preterm labor. She is no longer actively bleeding and, after the patient talks the midwife out of doing a speculum exam, the patient is released to go home with instructions to come back if the bleeding starts again.

It is important to note that for the majority of time Jennifer spends interacting with the patient, she is at the computer documenting her assessment and collecting updated patient information. She spent nearly the entire interaction attuned to the very real administrative pressure to document. She tells me that the cord to the computer in the triage room is so short that she cannot even face the patient while she documents. However, I notice that the cord is long enough that Jennifer could wheel the portable desk around to face the patient if she had wanted to. However, facing the patient is likely not a priority to her, an indication, again, of her process rather than patient orientation.

The next time I observe Jennifer is in November 2015, and her focus in January on the salary freeze turns out to have been prophetic. Jennifer has news: she is only working per diem now at Fuller, having taken a full-time job as an OB nurse in another hospital. She tells me that the financial pressures at Fuller pushed her over the edge: "Quite a few of us left this year because things have changed so much. One thing, I found myself to be making less money now than I was ten years ago." When I ask what she means, she explains:

Because they used to match our 403(b) contribution, and they took it away. . . . So, that's thousands of dollars that I'm not getting now, and our [health] insurance [premiums] went way up. It went to a high deductible plan, so that's a lot of money coming out of my pocket that wasn't a few years ago. And they kept promising a raise and taking it away, and yet the hospital administrator was constantly giving himself a Christmas bonus. You know, his pay is posted in the paper and, you know, [he gave] himself a 41 percent raise while we couldn't get the 3 percent raise we asked for.

She goes on to discuss how her job had become harder at the same time she was being compensated less:

Electric's gone up, food's gone up, gas has gone up, but my pay has actually gone down. But the workload has gone up. And then, when [the new obstetrics groups] started here, that was right after they told us we weren't getting any raises. What happened was, the union, that we pay almost eleven dollars a week to be a part of, negotiated and said, "You're going to get a 1.5 percent raise in April and a 1.5 percent raise in October, for a total of 3 percent, so hang in there." Okay, so six months go by. April comes around. The hospital says, "You know what, we don't have it, but we will give you the full 3 percent in October—not retroactive from April to October with the 1.5 percent, no—but we will give you the full 3 percent in October." The union agreed. Okay. So, October comes around, and then, all of the sudden, it was, "Nope, we don't have anything. You're not getting anything." So, no raise. Zip.

She goes on to say that the buyout by Axiom was "dangled" in front of the nurses, who were told that things would be better if they would only be patient.

Jennifer also brings up her assessment that danger has been introduced into patient care, and that this puts her at risk for being blamed. For example, she says, "If we're really busy . . . our licenses are on the line . . . We're talking about that kind of busyness." When I ask her to explain what she means by dangerous situations, she says:

Having too many patients or having to leave a patient under your care that doesn't have a room. And there have been times where we've had to say, "Oh my gosh! Can you just hang out here? We're waiting for the triage room to be cleaned. Somebody just left, and there's not a single other room." We've also had to put people in the OR recovery room, where, you know, you're trapped back there behind a locked door. There's no bathroom there for the patient. We started to feel like, if something bad happens, like the patient who had a stroke last year, if that happened now, when it was super busy, that would be . . . I don't even want to think about it. Who knows what the outcome could be? So, that really scares us quite a bit.

These conditions—financial concerns and liability risk—led her to leave a job she loved.

Recall, too, that Jennifer previously valued her job because it gave her a chance to socialize with other nurses. She tells me that now the hospital is so busy, those socializing times are limited if available at all. Jennifer laments, "It wasn't fun anymore to come [to work]." She says part of the problem is that, with so many new nurses and orientees, the nurses have to get together outside of work to socialize because there is hardly time to socialize at work anymore.

In fact, I was struck, in my post-March 2015 observations, how many new faces there were. It felt like a different unit. When I ask Jennifer about this she tells me:

Basically, the ones who still are here are the ones who are close to retirement and the new ones who wanted OB and finally they were able to get in because positions opened up. And those of us who are not close to retirement but have plenty of experience and are marketable, have gone. Because we found better paying, better jobs.

Patients do not benefit from losing nurses with experience, and it is the case that having many new nurses makes the unit fundamentally different.

I focus on Jennifer to illustrate the full impact of changes. She is a nurse concerned about documentation and following protocols. She worries about malpractice issues and losing her license. When the risks become too high and the financial pressures personally affect her, she finds another job.

Heather

Heather is a nurse who had a child at a young age and entered Fuller Hospital's OB unit as a new nurse, not long before I began my research. Like Jennifer, she left for another job following the upheaval surrounding Axiom's pullout.

Heather Pre-Axiom

It is a busy day and Heather is frustrated with a postpartum patient's request for help breastfeeding. As charge nurse, Heather is dealing with a staff shortage, which is why she has assigned herself a postpartum patient. When the patient "calls out" for breastfeeding help, Heather says, "Ugh!" and makes a face. But she goes to the room. Like many other process-oriented nurses, Heather does not embrace patient-oriented care, but the care takes place, though not enthusiastically.

In fact, not going above and beyond required protocols in the care of patients is a marker of a process-oriented nurse. During an observation in February 2014 Heather is assigned to a difficult patient. The patient has a history of domestic violence and what Heather characterizes as an unreasonable demand, which involves a restraining order the patient has against an unnamed individual. The patient does not want to disclose to the hospital the name of the person from whom the restraining order protects her. Rather, she wants the nurses to tell her the name of any visitors so that she can then decide whether they should be let onto the unit. This is an onerous demand for the nurses. Heather makes it clear that she is not happy with this request and repeats her dislike for the patient throughout the day, commonly referring to her as a "DCF [Department of Children and Families] train wreck." It was striking to me how patient characteristics are discussed in such a derogatory way, and this negative talk about patients was common among process-oriented nurses, perhaps because patient care is not their main focus. This allows for class biases to seep into care.

My analysis suggests that it is common for process-oriented nurses to be frustrated with patients, especially when they ask for extra help or have requests not in line with typical care. It is clear this tendency is exacerbated on busy days. However, it is important to note that busy days occur in the pre-Axiom period, but they are interrupted by days that are quite slow. As already discussed, that changes dramatically after the attempted takeover disintegrates.

Heather Post-Axiom

I observe Heather again in January 2015, just after Axiom pulled out of the acquisition. She is caring for a patient Evelyn had assisted the previous two days being induced for pregnancy-induced hypertension. Evelyn's care of this patient is documented in chapter 3. Heather's care of the patient differs markedly from Evelyn's. Although Heather is critical of the care the patient received over the past two days—calling it a "half-assed induction"—she does no more to progress the induction than Evelyn did and provides less direct care. Heather is rarely in the room except to turn up Pitocin and to take vital signs. She cares for the patient for her entire shift and makes sure to document everything precisely. However, she does little in the way of encouraging the patient or spending time with her.

She talks to me quite a bit about what she needs to do for the patient, and her discourse is mostly technical:

> I need to draw blood today because the blood count is only good for twenty-four hours. We need that if we're going to do a c-section. The IV should only be in three or four days. If it looks okay, we can leave it in, but you really have to get a special order to leave it in. If she has a c-section, she'll have an IV for twenty-four hours after that, and then you're sort of looking at an IV being in her arm a really long time.

Her technical discourse continues as she talks to the patient. For example, when she goes to the patient's room to give her a second IV to administer Pitocin, she tells the patient, "If you have Pitocin for a while with magnesium, it increases your chance of extra bleeding. So, it's good to have an extra IV site anyway." Compare this to the more encouraging pep talks and explanation given to patients by patient-oriented nurses. Note, however, that Heather does not get behind in her documentation the way patient-oriented nurses do. *Not* spending extended periods of time encouraging the patient gives her time to stay up on charting.

Other examples show how Heather provides care differently than do patient-oriented nurses. When Heather places the second IV, the patient is clearly anxious and in pain, as evidenced by her kicking her legs and feet and groaning. This is a situation in which Lillian, a patient-oriented nurse, likely would have broken into song or some other form of distraction. Heather does no such thing. When the patient says, "I hate needles," Heather responds by saying, "Well, if you liked them, that would be a problem. No one likes them. Well, I guess I've known a few people who like needles. Needles kind of suck. Lots of pressure. I'm sorry." She also fails to change the patient's sheets, although the night nurse had left out a fresh set and a new gown for the patient. Heather never offers to change the sheets or to help the patient into a new gown, things Evelyn went out of her way to do for this patient the day before. Further, Heather does not watch the patient when she walks to the bathroom. Evelyn always kept a watchful eye on the patient anytime she was up because magnesium makes patients "fuzzy." However, Heather simply asks the patient if she is okay, and when the patient responds positively she goes back to charting, no doubt documenting the patient's answer to her question.

In fact, Heather is so focused on charting that she does not always hear when the patient or her partner asks her questions. Further, her communication with the patient continues to be strictly technical. When the new physician on call decides to stop the patient's magnesium, Heather tells the patient, "Your risk of seizing is low." Heather's explanation of why the doctor is stopping the magnesium is quite technical, and my assessment of the situation is that the patient likely did not fully understand what Heather meant. A more patient-oriented nurse might have explained that the magnesium is being stopped because the patient's blood pressure is under control and she shows no other symptoms of preeclampsia, which nearly eliminates the risk of eclamptic seizure. A patient-oriented nurse might also have reminded the patient that magnesium relaxes muscles and makes it harder for the uterus to contract. Instead Heather tells the patient, "It [turning off the magnesium] will help you to deliver."

When Heather tells the patient that she will take out one of the IVs since she doesn't need magnesium anymore (and thus only needs one IV site) and asks her which IV is more annoying, the patient quickly answers the question by pointing her finger to one of the IVs; Heather responds, "Well, I'm going to leave both in for a little bit, but we will come back to take one out." Heather does not reflect on what it means to a patient not to follow through on an offer to reduce pain and discomfort. Instead, she turns to charting. Finally, she asks the patient if she likes the peanut ball (it is still in the room from the day before, when Evelyn brought it in). The patient says yes, but Heather doesn't offer the ball to her for use. She tells me at one point during her shift that she is worried the patient is talking about her. This puzzles her, but it is clear to me that her goals align with the process-oriented objectives of appropriate and consistent documentation, which take nurses away from providing the one-on-one attention patients may value and expect. In other words, Heather is in an organizational bind.

Heather, like Evelyn from chapter 3, who also cared for this patient, is forced to deal with the incessant constraints and changes rolling through the OB unit. It is a weekend day, and Heather needs to take blood she drew from the patient when she placed the second IV to the lab for a CBC (complete blood count) test, but there are no nurses available to watch her patient while she goes to the lab, and there are no volunteers on the weekend who might take the tube to the lab. Even on a relatively slow day, nurses are still scarce and nurses feel the pinch. Heather says, to no one in particular, "I have to go run the CBC down [to the lab], just started my lady on Pit . . . I need water, and I need to blow my nose." Then, before she can continue to look around for someone to keep an eye on her patient, a triage patient comes in—one they have been expecting—and Heather is the only person at the front desk and must admit the patient. She sits down and gets to work doing something secretaries typically do. In a short time, she also has to deal with further staff shortages in the pharmacy, whose staff had not restocked needed medications for the unit. In other words, all nurses, regardless of their orientation, have been greatly affected by the changes at the hospital. Ultimately, Heather left for a job she found more secure, gave her more autonomy and flexibility, and reduced her risk of liability.

Crystal

Crystal never planned on being a nurse. She had plans of military service as a career but, after being in the military for a few years, was dissuaded by her husband, who wanted her to stay in the United States to raise a family. Still, nursing was not anything she considered until she was with a military friend during her birth. She tells me:

> After my friend had a baby, I went back to school to become a nurse because I loved [being with her during her birth] so much. . . . So, then when I had my own son, I went to nursing school full-time. . . . From that point, when my friend had a delivery, I just, I never wanted anything else other than labor and delivery.

In terms of supporting patients, she indicates:

> I feel like I have to meet the patient where they're at. I think each patient has their own needs and wants, and as a nurse, I think . . . like a decoding, like what do they need, what do they want? . . . It's the little things I think help support the patient as well. The little things like holding their hand, supporting them when they've had a loss, being present . . . especially in labor, supporting them, helping them to breathe through contractions.

The interesting thing about Crystal's answer is that the other nurses do not think she is good at her job, and she is very focused on completing paperwork and monitoring patients. That is, her words do not reflect her actions, and I observed her countless time obsessing over paperwork and protocols. It was not uncommon for Crystal to panic over a chart she could not find or an electronic charting function that she could not figure out how to perform. In fact, one of the things other nurses talked about in hushed voices is that they do not want Crystal to train to be charge nurse, even though she has the required two years of experience. They simply do not trust her abilities.

Crystal Pre-Axiom

Crystal is clearly a process-oriented nurse. For example, I was startled in my observations of her care of patients by how often she checks their cervical dilation, how infrequently she encourages them to move or walk, and how she insists on IVs for every patient. These practices are not consistent with patient-oriented nursing because she treats all patients the same regardless of their wishes. Crystal describes her use of procedures to patients as natural and necessary. Of course, there is nothing natural about medical procedures, and they are not necessary for every patient. However, they do allow for easy documentation of the fetal heart rate, fluid intake, and cervical dilation, which is her overriding concern.

A particularly striking example of her nursing style is how Crystal treats a particular patient with a history of precipitous (fast) labors. The patient is "Group B strep positive," meaning that she has a Group B streptococcus bacteria vaginal infection. Although many women have such an infection, it is a concern in pregnancy because the baby can be infected during birth, leading to respiratory disease, general sepsis, or meningitis.[10] The typical treatment for pregnant women infected with Group B strep to prevent the baby's being infected with the bacteria is to give them two doses of penicillin intravenously over four hours, ideally during labor and before the baby is born. The patient has been brought in for an induction to prevent a precipitous birth but, upon arriving, nurses find that the patient has already begun labor on her own. The induction is called off and penicillin is started. The woman is adamant that she does not want pain medication. Given this, it is surprising that Crystal does not suggest movement, a birth ball, or walking to ease the patient's labor pain. Further, Crystal checks the patient's cervical dilation nearly every hour, a practice that allows her to easily document the patient's labor progress.[11] Crystal converses with the patient about the beauty of the snowy day and their shared love of game shows. Nonetheless, the patient is given little choice in her care, a hallmark of process-oriented nursing.

Crystal's process orientation also comes across clearly in her discussion with Jennifer later in the day. Crystal tells Jennifer, the charge nurse, that she does not want to go into the patient's room because she is afraid the patient will tell her that she feels pressure to push, an indication that the baby is ready to be born. The charge nurse, Jennifer, supports her on this decision, telling her not to go into the room so that the patient does not start pushing before the doctor arrives. This shows a coalition of two process-oriented nurses who are more concerned with protocols (in this case that the doctor must arrive for the delivery) than they are with helping the patient deal with contraction pain (the patient is unmedicated) and the urge to push.

The patient does not give birth before Crystal's shift ends, when Evelyn, a patient-oriented nurse I discussed in chapter 3, arrives and is assigned to care for the patient. As Crystal gives a patient report to Evelyn, it becomes clear that she understands that Evelyn is much more patient orientated than she is. When Evelyn asks if the patient has been out of bed, Crystal disingenuously reports that she offered to help the patient walk or use a birth ball but that the patient declined. This is not true. I watched Crystal care for this patient over her entire shift that day, and she only one time mentioned to the patient getting out of bed but ended the suggestion with the statement "Or you can stay in bed," hardly encouragement to get out of bed and move. Evelyn is clearly frustrated and, when Crystal finishes her report, immediately goes to the room to talk to the patient. This example highlights how these nurses' priorities differ and can therefore cause clashes between nurses.

Although Crystal's orientation might be construed as problematic— subjecting patients to many cervical dilation checks and then not checking on a patient who is nearly fully dilated so that any breach in protocol is not acknowledged or documented—she is helping to meet the administrative goals of the hospital. Her frequent checks of the patient's progress earlier in the day allowed for the physician to make a rational guess as to when the patient will deliver and not "waste" time sitting in the hospital waiting for a delivery. Further, if the patient pushed before the doctor arrived, under the administrative protocols, nurses might rationally decide it is better not to have that documented. In the case of a bad outcome, it would be very damaging to the hospital to have documented that the patient was pushing but no doctor was present for delivery. It is situations like these that indicate the very real contradictions between administrative protocols and patient care.

Crystal Post-Axiom

I interviewed Crystal in June 2015, several months after Axiom had rescinded its acquisition offer of Fuller Hospital. What she noted is how busy the unit had become:

We are busier, considerably busier. . . . I know they have staffing issues here, where certain shifts are less staffed . . . and so that makes it . . . very stressful for certain nurses. And I've picked up extra hours to help out on other shifts because they need it. They need help. So, we've tried to help each other out by picking up hours and stuff so that we can cover the numbers so that it's not unsafe.

While Crystal mentions that nurses try to help each other out by covering extra shifts, it was also clear to me that she and other nurses are frustrated that management expects them to do this. They ask why the burden of nursing shortages are put on their shoulders. In fact, some nurses became so frustrated that they stopped checking the group's Facebook page and responding to desperate texts for nurses to come in and help. Notice, again, the characterization of the unit as potentially "unsafe" for patients. This is a concern expressed quite often by process-oriented nurses.

Further, I note that in the pre-Axiom time, staffing allowed nurses to choose whether to go to a patient's room. After the Axiom acquisition fell through, the nurses became so stretched thin that their not going to a room of a patient may not have been intentional but might have occurred because nurses were given more and more patients.

Julie

Julie is a nurse on the margin of process and patient orientation. She is fun loving and her laugh is contagious. She jokes with her patients and enjoys a jovial rapport, which seems to make her what I have defined as a patient-oriented nurse. However, she is a rule follower and spends most of her time outside the patient's room, which is why I ultimately classified her as process oriented.

Julie came into nursing through her boyfriend's mom's suggestion. She did not know what she wanted to do after high school. She tells me in a January 2015 interview:

I always liked the medical care field, but didn't know what I wanted to do. My boyfriend's mother suggested I apply to the nursing program at [local university] because there were openings. I did and started school just two months later, something that wouldn't happen anymore. Now there are waiting lists.

She worked in another state on a med-surg unit and then in an ICU (intensive care unit). She and her family moved back to her hometown, and Julie worked for five years in the ICU of a nearby hospital before moving to Fuller, again in ICU, but through a temporary agency. When the hospital stopped using the temp agency to staff nurses, she found herself out of a job. Fortunately for her, the OB unit manager at Fuller Hospital knew her as a good nurse and offered her a job. That was more than ten years before this interview. She had applied for labor and delivery jobs a few times earlier in her career but was told she needed more experience.

Julie Pre-Axiom

I follow Julie in September 2013, just as the Axiom offer is coming to light. She is caring for a VBAC patient, a Chinese woman who has only been in the United States for one month ("right off the boat" is Julie's characterization of the family, which she shares a number of times throughout the day). The patient had a cesarean in China four years before for low amniotic fluid levels. Julie explains that they do not have the patient's medical records from her previous physician. "The records are on a slow boat from China," she jokes. The patient has not labored before, and, thus, Julie tells the father of the baby that this is like a first labor. The patient arrived in labor the night before for a scheduled induction, again for low fluid levels. There are no other family members in the country, and the nurse from the night shift allowed the patient's four-year-old to stay the night with her parents.

Julie arrives for her day shift and is assigned the patient. She goes into the room shortly after her shift starts and just before she wants to go and eat breakfast. Just after she arrives in the room, a resident comes in and introduces herself to the patient. This is a typical way the residents ingratiate themselves with patients with the aim of witnessing a birth. This happens often and is due to the residents' need to see a certain number of births in order to proceed in their residency. After the resident introduces herself to the patient, Julie tells the resident, "She's been suffering all night and [is] exhausted." At this point the father of the baby asks for medication for his wife (he means an epidural). Julie says that she will ask the midwife.

The patient is laboring with Pitocin while in the bed, a painful combination. Although Julie offers the patient a seat in the rocking chair, she does not offer telemetry or suggest walking around, something that would help the patient deal with pain. Process-oriented nurses are much less likely than patient-oriented nurses to suggest telemetry. Telemetry makes it harder to monitor the fetal heartbeat and the patient's contraction pattern because movement disrupts the placement of the tracking mechanisms. Note that Jennifer, earlier in this chapter, was frustrated with the difficult time she had monitoring her patient with telemetry and wished that she would stay in bed. This lack of suggested movement combined with the midwife's saying "no" to an epidural since the patient is only two centimeters dilated leaves the patient to experience pain with little help to ease her discomfort.[12] When Julie finds the patient is four centimeters dilated at 8:55 a.m., the midwife approves the epidural, which she receives about an hour later.

Missing equipment and shortage of equipment again are a concern. In Julie's case, she is called to be the second nurse for a delivery and finds essential equipment is not available. The second nurse is responsible for the baby. Just as the baby crowns, the patient's nurse yells, "Mec! Mec!" This means that there is presence of meconium in the amniotic fluid. Meconium is the baby's first stool; if inhaled, the baby may aspirate. This is a serious condition. When meconium is spotted, a nurse calls for a pediatrician to come to the room by calling out the warning "Mec!" When Julie hears the call, she immediately calls a pediatrician and starts looking for the intubation equipment. The goal is to suction the meconium out of the baby's airway before a deep breath is taken (usually with a cry). Julie looks horrified. The intubation equipment is missing. She yells into the phone that they need intubation equipment. The panic in Julie's eyes and voice are undeniable—lifesaving equipment is missing. Thankfully, the baby gives out a big cry. Once this happens, they do not suck the meconium out. It is too late, and, presumably, a crying baby is fine. In short, the cry indicates that the baby did not aspirate meconium. The potential crisis is averted.

My final pre-Axiom observation of Julie is in May 2014, during a time when the acquisition approval process is in full force but the staff has very little information about what will actually happen. I follow Julie on a day she is the charge nurse. Julie barely has a chance to sit down because the unit is so busy. The day before there had been a slew of deliveries, starting with a vaginal delivery at 7:08 a.m., an emergency cesarean at 7:25 a.m. for placental abruption (a very dangerous situation that, in this case, led to documented fetal distress), two more vaginal deliveries in the next hour, and another at 12:30 p.m. All those deliveries added to an already full unit such that there are eleven postpartum patients and several discharges that need to happen today.

I arrive at the hospital at 7:15 a.m., just as the day shift is starting, and begin following Julie at 7:50 a.m. In addition to being in charge, Julie has two mom-baby pairs. She visits the first pair, in room 4, a mom from the Philippines who talks to us about having volunteered at another nearby hospital to learn U.S culture when she immigrated fifteen years before. Julie is chatting with the patient when she realizes there is no blood pressure cuff in the room. She says, "Someone stole it from me. I knew I should have put it in the room so they couldn't steal it from me!" In the OR and in the triage rooms there is a blood pressure cuff and thermometer on the wall, but not in the LDRP rooms. Nurses have to find them. She continues, "The ironic thing here is that they're always about patient safety and patient satisfaction, but they always tell us they don't have the money—'We can't do this.'" She says that she particularly likes the carts with both a thermometer and blood pressure cuff but that there are only two carts and eight nurses, leading to constant competition over them. She finds a blood pressure cuff and completes the patient's assessment.

She then goes next door to her second mom-baby pair, in room 5. This patient is the talk of the unit because she delivered her baby the day before in her physician's office. She had called the office to tell them that she was cramping every five minutes. They told her to come in to the office to be checked. When they examined her, they found she was fully dilated. Her doctor decided to send her to the hospital in an ambulance, but when they called the OB unit at Fuller, the charge nurse informed them that there were no available rooms. The nurses tried quickly to clean a room and get it ready, but in the meantime the patient delivered in the office. Julie jokes with the patient, "You can have your baby at home, in the hospital, or (drum roll!) in the office!" She asks the patient whether the baby has been "eating" well (i.e., breastfeeding). The woman assures her that the baby has. Julie tells her that she will get her up after she eats breakfast and needs to perform tests after 12:30, when the baby is twenty-four hours old, including a hearing test and a cardiac test, both mandated by the state. As we leave, Julie asks if she needs anything. The woman asks for water and cranberry juice, and Julie leaves to retrieve them from the patient kitchen.

On the walk toward the kitchen, Julie tells me about how busy the day before had been. As she is talking we see a physician who says it was so busy yesterday that she cannot figure out which pharmacy she called with a patient's prescription. She can remember calling it in, but the pharmacy she thought she had called does not have a record of it. As we are listening to the doctor, Ashley, a nurse highlighted later in the chapter, comes in for a four-hour shift. She asks Julie, "What's the plan?" Julie tells her, "Just help everyone." She continues, "There's a cart; Rachel is having to do a car-seat test."[13] She is implying with her words and wave of a hand that Julie should do vitals on Rachel's patient. Julie turns and tells me, "A busy unit is okay if you have enough people."

Before we can get the water and cranberry juice to take to Julie's patient in room 5, a mini crisis occurs—a bilirubin meter is missing. This is a subcutaneous meter, which allows nurses to read bilirubin levels by scanning the baby's forehead rather than pricking the foot for blood. These meters are new and expensive—I attended a brief training class with a nurse on how to use the meters in an earlier observation—and nurses are not supposed to take them out of the nursery. The nurses are sure that Crystal has it, but they cannot find her. A mad chase for Crystal ensues, and she is eventually found and the bilirubin meter is recovered.

Then there is a loud crash. Julie runs to the back hall. She finds a staff member from engineering. He is standing on a ladder with a cart at his side. He says that he dropped some equipment and caused the crash. This crisis solved, Julie goes into the nursery to get an "advertising bag" (Julie's words). It has the hospital's name on the side and is a nice zipping canvas bag. She puts in information about breastfeeding, a box of Pampers diapers, and some Kleenex. She then goes to room 5 to give the patient the bag. The woman asks if it is okay that the baby has been nursing for thirty-five minutes. Julie tells her that it's fine but that there is a difference between the baby's nursing and the baby's using her as a pacifier. The patient says that the baby's nursing is starting to hurt her, and Julie tells her that it is fine to unlatch the baby. As she leaves the room, Julie tells the patient that the secretary is working on discharge papers and that she will bring them in when they are ready. Julie tells me outside the room that it is good to see the baby latched for so long because the baby had trouble "eating" last night. She still has not delivered the promised water and juice to the patient.

There is finally a bit of a break at 8:42 a.m., and Julie says she is going to eat her breakfast. She goes to the break room, where several people are sitting at the table. One, a midwife, tells how she heard that the woman who delivered in the physician's office yesterday was placed on a table without locking wheels. Thus, every time she pushed, the table ran over the nurse's feet. They all laugh about this. Jennifer asserts that she was so glad when they found out the baby was born in the office because they did not have room for her.

The secretary comes into the break room and asks Julie if she needs a nurse, Liv, to come in today.[14] Julie answers no because Ashley came in and Lillian is coming in at eleven. She thinks out loud about which patients are leaving and then tells the secretary, "No, we don't need her." Julie quickly finishes her breakfast and follows the secretary to the front desk to confirm her staffing. She walks back to the break room and asks Ashley if she can cover the baby at the scheduled cesarean at 9:30 because the NICU has five babies and, thus, a NICU nurse cannot cover the cesarean. Ashley reluctantly agrees.

Julie stays in the break room until 9:25 a.m., when she goes to the front desk to see if anyone has been discharged. Julie declares that she is happy there are so many baby girls because there are no circs (i.e., circumcisions) and, thus, discharges will be quicker. She says that she can discharge room 5 as soon as Tina, another nurse, finishes her charting. She tells me that sometimes women will ask if they can stay because they want to take a nap, and this patient did ask that. But there is no room. She tells me if the patient needs a ride, though, they let her stay.

A couple walks in with a days-old baby. The baby needs an outpatient bilirubin test, and the parents would like it done before they take the baby to the doctor for a scheduled visit. However, the baby is not in the computer system, so Julie has to call admitting. She then goes to the nursery to set up a warmer for the baby. She goes back to the main desk only to learn that Jennifer has just talked to a physician on the phone and agreed to admit for treatment a pregnant patient with an umbilical hernia. The physician wants to give her IV sedation and push the hernia back in. Julie is frustrated that Jennifer did not ask her to take the call, since she is in charge. She feels strongly that this procedure should be done in the emergency room and says that she would not have agreed to accept the patient, especially not on such a busy day.

She goes back to the nursery to perform the bilirubin test. She takes a Band-Aid off the baby's left foot, saying that she hates when people leave Band-Aids on babies. As she pulls the Band-Aid off, the secretary comes in the nursery and tells Julie, "This is crazy shit!" referring to the patient with the umbilical hernia who has been sent to the unit. Julie agrees and asks, "What happens if something goes wrong?" The secretary asks if the nurse manager knows about this, because "we can't do conscious sedation here." Julie tells her, "Well, Jennifer took the call and didn't ask me about it." Julie leaves the baby in the warmer and goes to talk to the nurse manager. The parents are not with the baby but waiting in the front hall, and I wonder what they would think if they knew that Julie had left the baby in the warmer, safe but alone.

She finds the nurse manager in her office, and Julie apprises her of the situation. Julie tells her, "I don't think we should do this. Do you think this is appropriate?" The nurse manager says, "No. This should be done at the ACS [ambulatory care center]. This doesn't make any sense. We can't do IV conscious sedation here." Getting the answer she wants, Julie goes back to the front desk and calls the physician to tell her that they cannot treat the patient in the unit. The physician tells her that the patient is already on her way to the hospital and that if they send her to the ER, the nurses in the OB unit will have to perform an NST (non-stress test) after she's treated. An NST is a test in which the woman is hooked up to fetal heart and contraction monitors for a designated period of time, usually about an hour, and observed.[15] Julie tells the physician that they will do the NST, clearly frustrated.

She goes back to the nursery and complains to three nurses about the whole situation. Julie pokes the baby's right foot, and he screams. Camila, a nurse helping Julie with the test, asks, "Did you give him any sucrose?" Julie answers, "No." Sucrose is commonly used to relieve neo-natal pain during procedures, and it is quite unusual at this hospital for sucrose not to be given during such a procedure.[16] Julie's not giving the infant sucrose is likely an oversight and an indication that she is doing too much and spreading herself too thin. Yet this is not her fault. She is in charge and dealing with a sticky situation, all while she still has patients assigned to her. Julie retrieves sucrose from a supply cart in the nursery and gives it to the baby, letting him suck it off her finger. He immediately stops crying. She finishes drawing the blood, bundles the baby back up, and takes him to his parents. She tells them that she will send the test results to the pediatrician. It is now almost 10:00 a.m.

Without a moment to spare, Julie immediately starts looking for the chart for the baby in room 5. She cannot find it, which slows the discharge of the patient. She finally finds it and heads to the room to ready the patient for discharge. She shows the patient how the top drawer under the crib has items she may take home with her, like nail clippers. She tells her to take everything in the top drawer. As Julie leaves the room, a custodian who works on the floor tells Julie to call downstairs because she needs help. The custodian says that there are three rooms to clean and "I can't do it all myself."

Julie goes to the front desk, calls the custodial department, and relays the request for help. She then goes back to room 5 to take the security tag off the baby.[17] As she walks into the room to do this, a family member is standing over the sink with a quizzical look on her face. She was washing her hands and a ring slipped off her finger and went down the drain. Julie tells her that she will call engineering to come up to retrieve the ring. The mom asks Julie about the lactation consultant. She has not yet been in to see her, and the mom is concerned about the baby's nursing for thirty-five minutes on one side. Julie tells her, "The baby's bilirubin is fine, sugar level is fine, and your baby is peeing and pooping, so she's getting milk. So don't worry!" Julie has not offered breastfeeding help, something most nurses would do since the patient has expressed breastfeeding concerns the last few times Julie was in the patient's room. Julie simply does not have time to deal with this noncritical issue. Thus, the patient is left to deal with the breastfeeding problem on her own.

Julie leaves the room, tells the secretary about the ring, and asks her to call engineering. The secretary responds by throwing her hands up in the air, exclaiming "If the ring is that loose, she shouldn't wear it!" She also informs Julie that the umbilical-cord patient is in the waiting room.

Julie asks the secretary for engineering's extension and then sits down to dial. Rachel, seeing Julie's exasperation, offers to call for her, and Julie readily accepts. Relieved from calling about the ring, Julie instead calls the OB practice of the umbilical hernia patient and talks to one of the physicians. It is just after 10:00 a.m. She explains that they are "popping at the seams, but the poor lady is here now." She says that it is a really busy day and that this procedure should have been scheduled at 3:00 or 4:00. She continues by saying that if the patient goes to the emergency department they will gladly do a non-stress test afterward. She hangs up. The physician from this practice who is on call and sitting at the front desk overhears the conversation. She tells Julie that she agrees that the patient should not have been sent to the unit. Julie seems relieved at this point that a physician in the practice agrees the patient should go to the emergency department, meaning that the patient will not take an LDRP room.

Having resolved that issue, Julie returns to patient care. She finally gets a pitcher of water and takes it to the patient in room 5. When she takes this into the room, the patient asks if there is a transparent disposable bag she can use. Julie tells her yes. She then goes to the supply room for the bag. Julie grabs it and takes it back to the room. She tells the patient that she will get the discharge paperwork as soon as she can.

Julie leaves the room and goes to the desk. She tells me that she needs to go and talk to the umbilical hernia patient to see if she wants to go to the emergency room. She walks to the OB waiting room, just outside the unit's door and near the elevators. There is a very pregnant woman sitting in the waiting room. Julie approaches her and explains, "We do not do hernia repairs on the floor," and tells her that she needs to go to the emergency department. The woman starts to cry. When she gets up from the chair to walk to the ER, she nearly collapses and leans against the wall for support. The woman is clearly in a great deal of pain. Julie, still insistent that the patient will walk herself to the ER, tells her how to get there. The patient starts to cry again. Julie, looking exasperated, tells her that she will walk her to the ER. Julie looks at me and says, "Who cares if they can't find me?" She's indicating the problem of leaving the unit as charge nurse.

The trip involves stairs and several turns, and I tell Julie that I could not have found the ER even if she had told me how to get there. We arrive at the ER, and Julie has the patient sit down while she goes to talk to the secretary. The problem: the secretary tells Julie they are not expecting the patient and that she will need to talk to her nurse manager. The secretary goes with Julie to talk to the nurse manager, who also says that she is not expecting the patient. Julie tells her that an obstetrician is going to come down to the ER to perform the procedure because they cannot do it in the OB unit. The nurse manager tells her that the patient has "at least an hour wait." Julie thanks her and leaves the ER without telling the patient or even saying good-bye. This was a difficult situation for me because I felt like I was participating in abandoning a patient. I regretted wearing scrubs and blending into the nursing staff. But I understood from Julie's perspective why she was leaving. She was in charge and was expected to be in the OB unit at all times during her shift. She is following protocol.

Julie arrives back on the unit at 10:30 a.m. and tells another nurse, Tina, what is happening with the umbilical hernia patient. They discuss this. Jennifer tells Julie that they received a phone when she was gone and that one of the practices is sending a patient over who may be in labor. The nurses start to discuss rooms, because they do not know where the new patient will go. The custodian is cleaning the only LDRP room open right now. In the face of these pressures, they learn that one of the practices has decided to admit a triage patient who is thirty-six weeks pregnant and has high blood pressure. The doctors will perform a cesarean over the weekend. Julie had been counting on having that room open. Thus, they now have two patients needing LDRP rooms and no open spots. I can feel the stress in the unit, and it is hard not to be empathetic to the situation. They leave the issue unresolved.

At 10:35 a.m. Julie goes to room 4 and checks the patient's vital signs. The blood pressure cuff is missing, and she leaves the room to get a cuff and a thermometer. While looking for these, Julie realizes she needs a stethoscope, too. She asks me, "Why is this so hard to find?" Before going back to the room, she realizes that she has not set the bed for a cesarean, a responsibility of the charge nurse. Thus, before she goes back to room 4 with the blood pressure cuff, thermometer, and stethoscope, she goes to set the bed. She finds a bed, and I help her to maneuver it to a position just outside the operating room. This is the bed the patient will be transferred to when she is done with surgery. She then puts the patient's belongings in bags and takes them to room 12, where the patient will be taken from the recovery room.

Finally, she makes her way back to room 4 with the appropriated equipment and goes to take the baby's temperature. But, alas, she finds that there are no probe covers. "Somebody should have replaced these!" she exclaims. She makes her way to the supply room to get the probe covers and goes back to the room. The patient is in the restroom and tells Julie that there are no more ice packs. Julie checks and finds that the patient is right. She sighs and goes back to the supply room once again to get more ice packs. She comes back into the room and takes the baby's temperature. While the patient is in the restroom, Julie tells her that she can take a shower anytime she wants and retrieves some soap from one of the drawers built into the cabinets in the room. She puts the baby in the crib and waits for the patient to come out. When she does, Julie turns to leave. As we walk out of the room together, Julie tells me, "I never say it's busy. I never tell patients that we have a busy floor. I only say that we're very popular today."

Needless to say, the day continues at this frantic pace, with room shortages, missing equipment, and the custodian being overwhelmed with cleaning rooms. This explains why, half way through the day, Camila says to no one in particular, "Days like yesterday and today are why the charge nurse shouldn't have two or three patients." Lillian agrees, saying, "You know, it's not uncommon in big hospitals [for] charge nurses [not to have] any patients."

The interesting thing to remember is that this observation occurs before the time of uncertainty around Axiom's taking away the acquisition offer. Further, the new OB practices had not started deliveries at the hospital yet. Even then there were definite stresses of room and staffing shortages. This was only to get worse over time with more patients. These terribly frantic and busy days happened before 2015, but they were not the norm. Note, though, that staff—custodial, engineering, and secretarial—are all available and working, and that nurses come in and help. Julie even turns down one nurse's offer to come in to help. Further, although rooms are "short," the custodian has help cleaning three rooms, meaning that these can be made ready for patients quickly. All of this changes after Axiom pulls its acquisition offer and makes the job of nurses much more difficult, especially on "busy" days.

Julie Post-Axiom

I interviewed Julie in September 2015, nine months after Axiom pulled out and just a few months since the hospital told the nurses that Waranoke's acquisition had been accepted. In the interview, Julie tells me how new nurses are being hired into the unit with little experience. I ask her why this is, as it is unusual for OB positions not to require a minimum of two years of experience in another unit, preferably medical-surgical. Julie tells me that experienced nurses are leaving and that the hires are necessary.

Julie is keenly aware of the effect of national policy changes on her work life at the hospital. She points out to me how patient satisfaction surveys, a policy promoted by the ACA, are important because they are "driving reimbursements." Julie is aware how the new policies have made it more difficult for her to take care of patients. She discusses both the increased patient load and the lack of resources.

I ask her about other changes, and she rattles off a laundry list: pay freeze, 401(k) employer contribution freeze, and increased cost of health insurance for nurses. She also tells me of the crunch in rooms, sharing stories of a patient laboring in a wheelchair in a tub room and another laboring in the waiting room because LDRP rooms were not available. She tells me that support staff have been cut and nurses have to fill in the gaps. She says, "I mop more, take out the trash more, and make up more rooms than I used to."

I ask if her list of issues developed during the time since Axiom stopped courting the hospital, and she confirms that it has. She ultimately blames the state for having put onerous constraints on the Axiom acquisition, a common sentiment among the nurses, who were typically not fans of the governor. I ask her if things are harder for nurses since Axiom pulled out of the acquisition. She says absolutely because the deal falling through led to budget constraints. She tells me that is when the "no raises" policy started. She continues by explaining that the hospital is losing money, which "comes out of our pockets." She also points out the issue of supplies and equipment being missing or low. She gives the example of diapers and wipes running out on the weekends and on holidays. She indicates that running low on supplies is also due to support staff being cut to save money. Thus, nurses have to fill in the gaps, performing duties like restocking.

She also suggests another indicator of "busyness." She says that in 2014 she had been called out 120 hours. That means that she had been placed on call (i.e., told that she did not need to work a scheduled shift) for 120 hours over the year. She said that since January 1, 2015 (nine months ago), she has been called out only twenty-four hours, not the commensurate ninety hours one would have expected based on her 2014 rate of being placed on call. She continues, "When there is a down day, which there hardly ever is anymore, if a manager sees nurses talking, that nurse will be told to 'get to work restocking or going through and throwing out old meds.'" She says that the unit has been so busy that the nurse manager has come in to help with deliveries at 4:00 or 5:00 in the morning and circulated in the OR. This is a definite change from even a few months earlier. Yet, working overtime is forbidden, which creates an incredible contradiction for the nurses because nurses are forever being called to come in to help. However, if their coming in puts them into overtime, they will be "talked to" about this. This is a clear bind for nurses that was not present just a few months earlier.

Ashley

I end with Ashley, perhaps the most process-oriented nurse on the unit. I begin this analysis of Ashley's behavior with an observation that illustrates well this orientation. "I don't like her," Ashley tells me, speaking about a patient she's caring for today. She continues, "It's just that it's nice when we have a nice loving family that deserves to have children. She's like a teenager!" The implication, of course, is that this woman does not deserve children. The woman's faults: she is young (early twenties), is obsessed with her phone, and her husband has recently been released from prison for a nonviolent criminal conviction. No doubt, it is hard to identify with such patients, but to allow one's dislike of such a patient to affect care is unconscionable. Jeanne Flavin writes about such attitudes and beliefs, which are deeply ingrained in our society, in her award-winning book *Our Bodies, Our Crimes*. Flavin argues that procreation is a human right and that those in positions of authority (e.g., physicians, judges, police officers, or, in this case, nurses) often confuse that right with the right to parent. Clearly Ashley is doing this.

Not only is Ashley condescending toward this patient, but she also taunts the patient in a way that may not be obvious to the woman. The patient is being induced for low amniotic fluid levels, a condition known as oligohydramnios. The midwife caring for the patient tells Ashley that the patient refuses to drink water, saying it makes her feel sick. Ashley makes it a point each time she leaves the patient's room to ask her if she wants water. Ashley is offering water to the patient *only* because she is aware that the patient has indicated that water makes her feel ill. Late in the morning, after having offered the patient water several times, Ashley tells the midwife that she keeps offering the patient water. She laughs at the joke she is pulling on the patient. I find it hard to witness this type of behavior. It is not about taking care of the patient in any way but about making fun of her. This is typical of her care of patients.

Ashley Pre-Axiom

Ashley emphasizes monitoring machines. This is typical of how process-oriented nurses behave in their care of patients. Ashley is orienting a new nurse one day, and she emphasizes to the orientee how to use the monitors. She says to the orientee while at the front desk, "You always want the uterine contraction monitor on because then you can see the uterine contraction in relationship to the fetal heartbeat." Yet, continuous monitoring of the fetal heartbeat, with or without a contraction monitor, raises a woman's chance of cesarean.[18] Thus, she is emphasizing a practice that increases the cesarean rate. However, note that this practice is in line with the organizational goal of preventing lawsuits. Continuous monitoring provides information that may allow a provider and hospital to avoid or to defend themselves in a lawsuit. I overhear an orientee later in the day say at the front desk, "The strip looks wonderful. I could just watch it all day." Process-oriented nurses are socializing new nurses in their way. I know of no better indication than a new nurse swooning over watching the strip. I say this because watching this strip means that she is not in the room caring for the patient.

I do not mean to suggest Ashley is not affected by change. She is, but she focuses on how she, herself, is affected. Other nurses experience this as making their work lives harder but also about how it makes it harder for them *to care for the patients.* Concern with patient care is not something that Ashley mentions in her interview or anything I saw in my observations.

Ashley Post-Axiom

Ashley is affected in a different way than perhaps other nurses are because she is only peripherally aligned with the goal of providing exemplary patient care. In November 2015 she is assigned a laboring patient. She is, as usual, at the desk during most of the day, this time shopping for American Girl doll clothes for her daughter. A resident wants to see her patient's birth, and he keeps hanging around the desk when Ashley is there, hoping not to miss it. He says to Ashley several times, "I just don't know the timeline of this." She finally tells him, "I wait 'til they're falling out. It saves our work and theirs. You know what I mean?" I use this as an example for her lack of patient orientation. I do not support such practices as coached pushing and strong directives in the second stage of labor; however, nurses typically stay in the room when patients are fully dilated, even if they do not coach pushing, to offer support and encouragement. The fact that Ashley is sitting at the desk shopping when her patient is fully dilated shows her lack of attention to patient care.

Ashley is at the far end of the spectrum in terms of her care of patients—she does the basic minimum and makes sure it gets charted—and because of this she is not the perfect example of a process-oriented nurse. But she is more process oriented than patient oriented because she focuses much more on documentation than on caring for patients. Her care is affected to the extent that documentation pressures are more onerous due to more patients, and when she is in charge she similarly feels the pressure. I observed her being harsh with other nurses and coming close to tears when she was in charge in the post-Axiom period. But because she spends so little time on patient care, she is less affected by change than are other nurses.

It is important to note, too, that not all process-oriented nurses are as crass as Ashley is toward patients. Process-oriented nurses are more likely than patient-oriented nurses to ridicule or make fun of patients; however, the degree to which Ashley does this is not common. My point is that process-oriented nurses may be vulnerable to this type of loathing of patients *because* they value documentation and rule following more than they do patient care.

Conclusion

Process-oriented nurses promote hospital goals by focusing on rules and protocols. They experience stress when they cannot meet those rules. It is not that they do not care for patients. They do. However, they are much more likely than are patient-oriented nurses to internalize the belief that rules are there for a reason and that following those rules promotes the care of patients. The stress of organizational change causes all nurses to shift toward administrative goals, and this is evident in all nurses.

I remind the reader that I do not mean to demonize or to morally judge these nurses. Process-oriented nurses are fulfilling goals that are important to the hospital—following protocol and trying to prevent lawsuits. These are just not goals that nurses are typically thought to promote. Nurses may be judged through a gendered lens of expected nurturing behavior. Thus, when nurses focus on documentation and protocol more than on patient care, part of what may seem judgmental is that I document how these individuals don't fulfill the expected and gendered behavior of nurses.

PART III

The Root of the Problem

5

Health-Care Policy Changes and
Organizational Crisis

> Going forward in order for any . . . smallish hospital system to do
> well, they need to combine with others to be bigger, to have bet-
> ter purchasing power, and to be more efficient. . . . So, you're seeing
> that. You're seeing it all over, and it doesn't mean that a hospital has
> done poorly. It just means that this is . . . how the economy is, what
> you have to do to stay in good shape. (Pauline, Fuller Hospital OB
> administrator)

In this chapter I discuss sweeping changes in national and state
health-care policy as a way of understanding why Fuller Hospital
was thrown into uncertainty and sought acquisition. Drastic change
in policy occurs periodically in the United States. The extensive
national policy change associated with the period of study covered
in this book, July 2013 to June 2016, is the Patient Protection and
Affordable Care Act, more typically referred to as the Affordable
Care Act (ACA) or "Obamacare." The ACA created a fundamentally new environment for hospitals. Fuller had not only the ACA
to contend with, but also state-level policy changes that affected
hospital funding. What we know from organizational theory is that
managers and administrators try to deal with organizational uncertainty to promote their organization's survival and longevity. I can
say unequivocally, having interviewed hospital administrators and
completed research for this book, that the ACA and state-level policy
changes created an inordinate amount of uncertainty for Fuller Hospital. Thus, we should not be surprised that non-profit hospitals like
Fuller are being bought up by for-profit hospital systems at a quick
clip. Such changes, from the perspective of organizational theory, are
to be expected. This chapter summarizes the federal and state policies that affected Fuller Hospital.

The ACA, a.k.a. Obamacare

The ACA attempts to improve the U.S. health-care system by focusing on three aims: better care, affordable care, and healthy people / healthy communities.[1] The ACA has a two-pronged strategy to meet these aims—increasing health insurance coverage in the United States and reforming the health-care delivery system. Here I focus on reforms to the health-care delivery system because this strategy is tied more to the overall research question of this book, although there is clear overlap in how ACA programs affect both goals.

The ACA's attempt to reform delivery of health care is both complex and ambitious. In fact, some researchers have criticized it as having "too many divergent experiments and lack[ing] a coherent strategy."[2] This divergent and contradictory strategy is due to the many compromises forged during the writing of the ACA.[3] Although detailing the compromises is explored well by Paul Starr and is beyond the scope of this book, it is important to note two things.[4] First, the compromise the White House and Senate Finance Committee made with the major hospital associations, in which the hospitals accepted reduction in Medicare and Medicaid payments, saving the government an estimated $155 billion over ten years, and in return were promised increased revenue due to the expansion of health insurance, did not affect all hospitals equally.[5] For example, the quality program that linked Medicare reimbursement rates to "appropriate" readmission rates (discussed below) was affected less by the quality of care provided in the hospital and more by patient and hospital characteristics, with non-profit hospitals losing on this measure because they typically have higher readmission rates.[6] Second, health insurance companies are the big organizational winners of the ACA, accumulating record profits since its rollout.[7] It is important to keep these caveats in mind throughout this chapter as one considers how hospitals respond to changes spurred by implementation of the ACA.

In reviewing the ACA, I follow David Blumenthal, Melinda Abrams, and Rachel Nuzum in their presentation of the changes the legislation has targeted: (1) changes in payment; (2) changes in the organization of health-care delivery; and (3) changes to make the government more responsive and flexible.[8] I focus here on the first two of these targeted changes because they are the changes that most affect day-to-day hospital decisions.

It should be noted that most of the policies dealing with reforming the delivery of health care apply to Medicare and, in a more limited way, Medicaid spending. This is because the government is the payer in these programs; thus, focusing on them is the easiest way for the government to affect health-care delivery and spending. Further, because baby boomers are now Medicare eligible, Medicare spending will cover a larger share of the population. However, although ACA policies focus on Medicare and Medicaid recipients, these policies are often based on private-sector programs and/or are adopted by health insurance companies in the private sector. Thus, the effects are not confined only to Medicare and Medicaid payment and services.

Changes in Payment

PAY-FOR-PERFORMANCE PROGRAMS

There are three pay-for-performance programs in the ACA, sometimes called P4P programs.[9] First, the ACA created the Medicare Hospital Readmission Reduction Program (ACA Section 3025). Beginning in October 2012, this program reduces hospital Medicare payments by 1 percent to hospitals that have higher-than-expected thirty-day readmission rates of Medicare beneficiaries for heart attack, heart failure, and pneumonia, as compared to national averages and adjusted for patient population. Since the beginning of the program, Medicare readmission rates have dropped by more than 19 percent.[10] Yet, some scholars feel that this program does not go far enough because it does not reward hospitals that have lower readmission rates, which would be a more comprehensive incentive for hospitals than just enforcing penalties.[11] Others dispute the implementation of the program and worry about using a thirty-day readmission rate and focusing on only a handful of conditions.[12]

An administrator of the OB unit at Fuller Hospital, who also had higher-level administrative responsibilities and was quite familiar with the ACA policies affecting hospitals, worries about hospitals being punished for higher than average readmission rates:

> They are just changing the entire way that people get paid . . . in terms of . . . not paying for certain services. . . . You have a patient who comes

in for pneumonia. If that patient is readmitted anywhere else within thirty days, not just for pneumonia—this is where the difficultly lies—if they are readmitted for any other reason, you don't get paid. . . . It's that kind of stuff, where you don't get paid for things that you reasonably should get paid for, and there's no other way for organizations to make money.

In other words, the Fuller Hospital administrator is focused, like some critics, on the ACA's emphasis on a small number of specific outcomes and its use of a punishment-based model, and also on the uncertainty created by the policy.

Second, hand in hand with the initiative to reduce Medicare readmissions is the ACA initiative to reduce hospital-acquired conditions, one of the causes of hospital readmission, through the Payment Adjustment for Hospital-Acquired Conditions Initiative (ACA Section 3008). Hospitals that are in the bottom quartile in terms of rates of hospital-acquired conditions lose 1 percent of their Medicare payments. The Department of Health and Human Services documented a 17 percent decline between 2010 and 2013 in the composite rate of hospital-acquired conditions, although it is not clear that this decline can be attributed to the ACA.[13] Fuller is one of the hospitals that was penalized for a high infection rate in both 2015 and 2016.[14]

Third, one of the most noted pay-for-performance programs tied to the ACA is the one I highlighted in the introductory chapter of the book: Hospital Value-Based Purchasing (VBP) (ACA Section 3001[a]). This program ties quality and cost of care to payment such that 1 percent of total Medicare payments for inpatient stays are redistributed to those hospitals that perform well on cost and quality measures.[15] The quality measures come from the HCAHPS survey.[16] The percentage of Medicare payment redistributed increased by 0.25 percent each year until it reached 2 percent in 2017.[17] This program is tied to nursing care because research indicates that nursing care has the largest impact on hospital HCAHPS scores, and nursing researchers advocate using measures of nursing care in any value-based purchasing program.[18]

A Fuller Hospital administrator told me in an interview about the problems she felt VBP presented for hospitals:

When value based purchasing first came out . . . it was very quick that we were able to get to a place where clinically we were meeting or exceeding the measure. But, in terms of what that meant for us as an organization in reimbursement, it basically was just like, "Okay, you've done that. Now you get to keep the money we've always been giving you." Instead of saying, you know, "You've gone above and beyond."

In short, this administrator identified the problem of asking hospitals to improve performance but with no additional compensation, just the threat of losing money. To receive any redistributed Medicare funds, the hospital must overachieve on both quality and cost measures, a tough task. Another unit administrator emphasizes the problem with using patient satisfaction surveys to determine payment: "They're holding our money until we meet certain requirements, like getting a high enough score . . . for example on our HCAHPS scores. If they are not high enough . . . they hold money in reserve. . . . It's money that is owed to us but we don't get it if we don't meet certain requirements." From a hospital administrator's perspective, this represents a significant challenge and a new, more competitive environment. Further, it is an uncontrollable dependence in the organization; ideally, organizations would minimize such dependences.[19] Health policy researchers suggest that the VBP program is the largest quality improvement program Medicare has ever introduced.[20] The contradiction for Fuller Hospital OB nurses, of course, is that patient satisfaction surveys matter most in an era in which their time with patients is crunched and they have trouble delivering adequate care.

I attended an OB meeting in 2016 in which the nurse manager discussed a new program that would follow up with new mothers over the phone to see if they need any help. She described this as "circl[ing] back to close the loop to make sure everything is okay." She indicated that the call would take only five minutes and it would not have to be done by a nurse but rather one of the unit administrators. She said that she had created a binder organized by the day the patient was discharged to make this easy to do. The benefit, she told the group, is that this is a nice way to see how services are going. If there is an issue, the card associated with the patient is flagged, and she (the nurse manager) can do a "customer service triage." She asked, "Why not do this? After all, car dealers call the next day to see how the service was; why shouldn't we?"

I was astounded at this discussion because the unit administrators and nurses are already taxed to such an extent that nurses are calling the unit unsafe. The nurse manager has been required to take furlough days, and the other unit administrators have attempted to fill in the gaps, although they tell me this has been impossible to do well. Unit administrators are already tasked with more than they can do. Triaging customer service should deal more with providing care, not trying to smooth over poor care after it happens. I have a hard time believing that nurses or unit administrators have time to make these calls. They are already stressed for time, and doing so will only take them away from patients more than they already are. There is no doubt, based on the conversation in the meeting, that this new program is an attempt by OB unit administrators to improve HCAHPS scores.

BUNDLED PAYMENTS

Another change in payment structure allows hospitals (as well as physician organizations and post-acute care providers) to participate in the Bundled Payments for Care Improvement initiative (ACA Section 2704). Bundled payments work through a single payment to a set of hospitals, post-acute care providers, and physician organizations for services that they provide to a patient for a given procedure or condition.[21]

The key to understanding bundled payments is to recognize that the focus is on an episode of care, or "the managed care provided by a health care facility or provider for a specific medical problem or condition or specific illness during a set time period."[22] This care may be provided in hospitals, medical practices, or post-care facilities. Thus, the focus is on providing care in a system. As an example, here's how the spending for episode of major joint replacement breaks down: inpatient stay at a hospital—50.9 percent; physician—11.9 percent; post-acute care—32.6 percent; readmission—3 percent; and other costs—1.6 percent. In other words, the care the patient receives for the *episode* of major joint replacement is bundled and *shared* among the hospital, physician, and post-acute organization. This program moves medical care away from focusing only on the care provided *at the hospital* and encourages hospitals to work in Accountable Care Organizations (discussed below) or to bring outpatient services within their hospital systems. The ACA bundled-payment program is a voluntary pilot program, which began in April 2013 and was expanded in October 2013.[23]

A hospital administrator discussed the effect of bundling payments on consolidation:

> Bundled payments, where there is only X amount of money and everybody who cares for the patient has to share that [money], instead of each group being able to bill themselves, that is what told the board and the senior leadership that they needed to become part of a larger network so that all of the services could be provided within, you know, a single network. Because any piece that you can't provide, then somebody else is getting part of that pie, that financial pie.

In other words, hospital administrators are attuned to the effect of changes in the funding of health care brought about by the ACA. Because administrators have focused on getting as many pieces of the pie as possible, this strategy explains their decision to seek out consolidation of physicians, hospitals, and post-acute care providers.

Changes in the Organization of Health-Care Delivery

As might be clear from above discussion, certain changes to health-care delivery might seem inevitable, particularly the industry's consolidation. Beyond this push toward consolidation, the ACA provides a pull, too—the means for consolidation.

ACCOUNTABLE CARE ORGANIZATIONS

One of the most noteworthy aspects of the ACA is its creation of Accountable Care Organizations, established by Section 3022. ACOs are defined as a group of providers who take on the care of a designated population within a certain budget. The ACO must have enough primary care professionals in order to provide care for at least five thousand patients and must also be able to report on measures of quality and cost.[24] ACOs are responsible for both the cost and the quality of care delivered to their designated population.[25] They are intended to "promote integration and coordination of ambulatory, inpatient, and post-acute care services."[26] The spending targets of ACOs are tied to the baseline Medicare spending for the designated population and projected forward on the basis of average increases in national Medicare spending.[27] National Public Radio produced a program on ACOs and explained them this way:

> Think of it as buying a television, says Harold Miller, president and CEO of the Network for Regional Healthcare Improvement and executive director of the Center for Healthcare Quality & Payment Reform in Pittsburgh. A TV manufacturer like Sony may contract with many suppliers to build sets. Like Sony does for TVs, Miller says, an ACO would bring together the different component parts of care for the patient—primary care, specialists, hospitals, home health care, etc.—and ensure that all of the "parts work well together."[28]

Although the ACA introduced the concept of ACOs for Medicare and Medicaid patients, ACOs have spread to commercial payers, such as health insurance companies.[29] The incentive for ACOs is that reimbursements are tied to both the cost of treating a patient and to quality of care measures, such that if costs are lower than a benchmark, the ACO shares the cost saving with Medicare, and in some programs if costs are higher, the ACO is assessed a penalty.[30]

The growth of ACOs has been tremendous. As of the end of January 2016, there were 838 active ACOs covering an estimated 28.3 million people in the United States.[31] These numbers indicate a significant growth in both measures—ACOs and people covered by ACOs—and ACOs exist in all fifty states.[32] One prediction is that ACOs will cover 70 million people by 2020 and 150 million by 2025.[33] ACOs are also quite diverse in terms of organizations that come together to form an ACO and populations that are covered.[34] As I demonstrated in the excerpt that started this book, hospital administrators see forming or joining ACOs as key way to navigate changes brought about by the ACA. As a reminder, the Fuller Hospital administrator told me, "I very firmly believe that community hospitals have to have that affiliation with a larger entity in order to be able to survive in the 'accountable care' kind of world." Nevertheless, for hospitals to become part of an ACO, they must make large investments in "consulting services, new information technology, utilization management tools, and management support" so that they can meet the demands of the ACO model.[35]

CHANGE IN CRITERIA FOR NON-PROFIT HOSPITAL STATUS

Another significant change to health-care delivery affects hospitals with a non-profit status. The ACA mandates new rules for hospitals to maintain non-profit status. Researchers have suggested that these new requirements represent a pushback from legislators who believe some non-profits are simply for-profit hospitals in disguise, with both providing charity work but only non-profit hospitals having the benefit of tax-exempt status.[36] According to analysts, the new requirements for hospitals to keep their non-profit designation are rigorous and expensive to institute and will likely have unintended consequences.[37]

The effect of the ACA on non-profit hospitals may not be evident because only one section of the legislation (9007) addresses this issue. Rather, the changes come from the application of the Internal Revenue Code §501(r), which creates new conditions a hospital must meet to continue to qualify for tax exemptions.[38] The four new conditions specified by the legislation are as follows:

1. Establish written financial assistance and emergency medical care policies.
2. Limit amounts charged for emergency or other medically necessary care to individuals eligible for assistance under the hospital's financial assistance policy.
3. Make reasonable efforts to determine whether an individual is eligible for assistance under the hospital's financial assistance policy before engaging in extraordinary collection actions against the individual.
4. Conduct a community health needs assessment (CHNA) and adopt an implementation strategy at least once every three years. (These CHNA requirements are effective for tax years beginning after March 23, 2013.)[39]

Beyond these new requirements, the ACA also added Section 4959 to the IRS code, which imposes an excise tax ($50,000 per hospital) for a charitable hospital's failure to meet CHNA requirements.[40] Further, if a hospital's CHNA shows that the community does *not* need its charitable care, the hospital will lose its tax-exempt status. This is problematic because it is unclear how the assessments should be performed and how the enforcement will happen.[41]

A less-considered effect on non-profit hospitals is the ACA-mandated reduction in federal Disproportionate Share Hospital (DSH) payments to hospitals that serve a large number of Medicaid and low-income, uninsured patients (ACA Section 3133). The reduction in DSH payments began in fiscal year 2018 (although it was to have begun in 2014, the change was delayed by legislation) with a $500 million decrease, and continues through 2020 with an aggregate $3 billion decrease.[42] The actual impact of this policy change is that beginning in fiscal year 2018 hospitals receive 25 percent of the amount they would have received under the previous DSH statute, with the remaining 75 percent payment available for uncompensated care payments, reduced by changes in the percentage of people who are uninsured.[43] The reasoning for this change is that with more people having insurance, DSH payments will not be necessary to provide care to people at the margins of society. Yet, health providers worry because hospitals still have to serve people who are the least likely to be insured, such as individuals who are addicted to drugs, mentally ill, or undocumented immigrants, and hospitals will now have reduced federal dollars to provide care.[44]

Medicaid compensation is a particularly sore spot for hospital administrators who, even though they know the benefit of the spread of Medicaid to more people, see the negative consequences to their hospitals because Medicaid reimbursements are low. This pressure is high on the mind of one of the unit administrators I interviewed:

> How do you keep reinvesting in your organization when . . . there aren't the dollars out there? . . . They've expanded Medicaid under the Affordable Care Act so more people are eligible. That's magnificent. That is wonderful. [But] Medicaid pays us about seventy-seven cents for every actual dollar of cost that we incur. . . . Medicare pays us, I want to say, ninety-one cents for every actual dollar. . . . So, we lose huge amounts of money with Medicare patients and especially with Medicaid patients. . . . So, in the past all the private insurances have needed to make that up. They've

needed to pay more. They've needed to pay us . . . $1.25 for every dollar that we have incurred. But now they don't want to do that anymore. They don't want to take on that burden. . . . So, they're looking to reimburse similar to what Medicare reimburses. And, again, there's this mismatch of then, who pays for it? And now that we have more people . . . receiving health insurance, we've got more people in the Medicaid pot, but even some of the health exchange plans, the reimbursement is so poor that some of the physicians aren't accepting those plans at all. . . . Doctors can choose that, but hospitals can't. Hospitals have no ability to say, "We're not going to take you."

The impact of these changes is difficult to ascertain, although many feel that the new requirements are onerous, especially for small, non-profit hospitals, for several reasons. First, the requirements are ambiguous.[45] For example, the regulation does not specify a dollar amount that hospitals must spend on charitable care.[46] Second, the Internal Revenue Service found that non-profit hospitals have a smaller operating margin to absorb these new regulations than do for-profit hospitals, which do not have to meet the new requirements.[47] Horwitz also suggests that small hospitals are hit the hardest.[48] In the pre-ACA time period of 2009 and 2010, small hospitals reported that a lower percentage of their total expenses were paid by means-tested government programs than did medium and, especially, large hospitals.[49] Third, others point to the difficulty imposed on non-profits by increased scrutiny and the threat of hefty fines for violations.[50] As a result, some suggest that the ACA will cause a fundamental realignment of the hospital industry toward for-profit hospitals.[51] As Gold writes:

> Cash-poor non-profit hospitals, unable to borrow money for needed improvements in facilities and equipment, are eagerly seeking for-profit suitors. And for-profit hospital companies and investment firms—eyeing the improving economy and the expected influx of millions more insured Americas as a result of the new federal health overhaul law—see opportunity in the non-profit sector.[52]

There are several examples of for-profit hospitals and hospital systems' buying not-for-profit hospitals, and the number of for-profit hospitals in the United States increased 38 percent between 1975 and 2012, with a 7 percent increase between 2009 and 2013, evidence of the continuing trend encouraged by the ACA.[53] Although the new requirements present hospitals a good opportunity to demonstrate their integration with their communities, for many hospitals these changes will be difficult to implement and represent a fundamental realignment of thinking.[54]

The ACA's Effect on Hospitals

Overall, the ACA has changed the mood of the country and, no doubt, this affects how hospital administrators and clinicians make decisions. Blumenthal, Abrams, and Nuzum sum this up eloquently when they write, "The provisions in the ACA regarding delivery-system reform have reinforced the impression that Americans are determined to bring health care costs under control and that providers would be well advised to help guide that process."[55] They argue that one of the administrative goals of the Centers for Medicare and Medicaid Services is for alternative payment mechanisms to cover 30 percent of Medicare payments by 2016 and 50 percent of Medicare payments by 2018, reinforcing this type of understanding by administrators and clinicians.[56]

The fact that the ACA has resulted in both symbolic and real changes in hospital reorganization is clear, as is significant potential for future change. For example, more than half of the cost reductions to health care through the ACA take place through cuts in Medicare spending.[57] The result of this might be a reduction in the number of hospitals, because hospitals may not be able to weather significant decreases in Medicare and Medicaid hospital spending.[58] Further, the merger incentive for non-profits may be extended to hospitals in general. Speculation is that the ACA is causing more hospital mergers, leading to "supersized" hospitals.[59] It is argued that size allows for the reduction in costs of many activities, such as billing and investment in electronic medical systems.[60] Another benefit of larger hospitals is that they may be able to negotiate higher prices with health insurance companies.[61] The hospital industry in the U.S. became markedly concentrated through the 1990's hospital merger wave such that by 2003, 88 percent of all residents living in a metropolitan area lived in a zone of high hospital concentration.[62] The structure of Accountable Care

Organizations is likely to increase concentration of the hospital market by bringing together hospitals and physician groups that otherwise would have been competitors.[63]

This leads to another effect of the ACA: physicians and hospitals are being pushed and pulled together in ways not common before the ACA.[64] There is the push of the ACA toward Accountable Care Organizations, which guides hospitals and physicians to establish new relationships. Scholars suggest that the focus on value-based purchasing and bundled payments gives physicians and hospitals incentives to work more collaboratively to decrease costs and increase quality of care.[65] However, this integration will not be easy and is not universally embraced by physicians or hospital administrators.[66]

Lastly, it must also be recognized that many of the ACA effects I have highlighted fundamentally focus on a realignment of the health-care delivery system, and this affects hospitals. For example, Devers and Berenson write that "developers of the ACO concept also emphasize accountability [like the health maintenance organizations developed in the 1990s], but focus directly on health care providers and the delivery system instead of insurers and HMOs."[67] This is different from earlier health-care reforms, which focused on insurers and HMOs rather than hospitals.[68] In other words, the fundamental difference of the ACA health-care reforms compared to earlier efforts is that the hospitals and clinicians are much more affected by the ACA changes.

The ACA is an example of swift national change to the health-care industry. Hospitals are affected by such change. But, it is important to remember that hospitals have at least two levels of regulators: national and state. Fuller Hospital was affected not only by national policy but also changes at the state level. The second part of this chapter will focus on those state-level reforms.

State-Level Policy Changes

The ACA and State Policies Spur Fuller's Quest for "Affiliation"

Fuller Hospital's troubles began with a combination of ACA policies and changes in the state tax policy. In the 2011 session, the state General Assembly passed a Hospital Net Patient Revenue Tax Act, effective July 1, 2011, which introduced a new tax on hospitals.[69] The governor suggested that the tax would raise $350 million from the state's hospitals. However, that sum (plus an additional amount) would then be redistributed back to the hospitals because the hospital tax would allow the state to take advantage of a Medicaid formula that rewards states that charge providers (i.e., hospitals) fees to help defray costs of caring for uninsured and poor patients.[70] Hospital administrators were skeptical from the start, which was warranted, as between 2011 and 2016 the tax on hospitals increased from $350 million in 2012 to $556 million in 2016, while the reimbursement to hospitals decreased from $400 million in 2012 to $60 million in 2015.[71] Thus, the net tax rate went from −$50 million in 2012 to +$496 million in 2016.[72] This is the tax to which the CEO of Fuller Hospital referred at the open meeting (detailed in the introduction of the book), when he discussed the state tax on hospitals that had negatively affected the hospital. No doubt, these state policy changes contributed to Fuller's financial woes.

At the same time, the ACA put increased financial and performance pressures on hospitals because payment structures changed. Fuller Hospital submitted a Certificate of Need (CON) application to the state in October 2015. This document gives us a glimpse into why the DHN board of directors sought an acquisition and the steps they took to do so. There is no doubt that DHN saw the ACA and state-level policy changes as threats. For example, in the CON application, DHN wrote:

> The adoption of the Patient Protection and Affordable Care Act ("PPACA") in 2010 further changed the landscape for health care providers, including [DHN], with significant planned reductions in government payments for services and requirements to participate in new payment models with a focus on collaboration and coordinated care.[73]

The application continues, "Then, in 2011, [state] reinstituted the hospital tax, putting an even further strain on [DHN's] finances. The combination of these factors led to the Board's decision to consider affiliation options."[74]

DHN quickly experienced financial crisis. At the end of the 2011 fiscal year, the first year of the hospital tax, DHN reported a "bottom-line loss" of $1.3 million.[75] This was at least partly due to revenue loss from the state hospital tax, which amounted to $580,000 in the fourth quarter of 2011 and $2.3 million for fiscal year 2012. According to the CNA prepared by DHN, in 2011, the network began to project how the organization would be affected for the next five years. The projection was worrisome: net revenues were projected to decline by $11 million per year, and operating losses of $6 million per year were expected. According to DHN, "These significant financial challenges led [DHN] management to conclude that future financial viability would require partnering." In the language of theories of organizational change, DHN was focused on regulation changes and changes to payment, which threaten its survival.[76] According to the theory, this should lead to action by DHN, and indeed it did. The weakening financial indicators of the hospital also indicate that bargains the Obama administration made with the hospital associations in order to pass the ACA did not help all hospitals.

The DHN board of directors established the "Partnering Workgroup" to "study the impact of PPACA on DHN and to evaluate whether benefits could be realized by affiliating with another health care system, or whether DHN would better serve the community by remaining an independent system."[77] The Partnering Workgroup shared its findings with the DHN Board in September 2012. The group concluded:

> Affiliation with a larger health system would better position [DHN] to achieve the following goals: (i) attract patients and providers based on quality, service, accessibility and affordability; (ii) enhance physician retention and recruitment; (iii) improve DHN's financial position in order to invest in new equipment and technologies; and (iv) coordinate care to manage risk and participate in new payment vehicles.

Notice that the fourth goal pertains directly to new payment methods implemented by the ACA. The group also put forth a list of potential for-profit and non-profit partners. The hospital board voted to pursue an acquisition.[78]

The board sent requests for proposals (RFPs) to six health systems (three non-profit and three for-profit), and four of the six indicated their interest—only one of them non-profit. By July 2013 the board had decided to pursue negotiations with Axiom.[79]

State Law Stands in the Way of Affiliation

However, state law presented a hurdle to the Axiom takeover. As a way of preventing the collusion of physicians and hospitals to charge higher fees, state law forbid for-profit hospitals from employing physicians. Because DHN owned physician practices (i.e., the hospital paid the salaries of those physicians and the costs of the practices) and employed hospitalists (physicians who only work in the hospital), this law presented a problem for any for-profit suitors. Further, because as many as four other non-profit hospitals in the state were considering for-profit acquisition partners, this issue became an important state policy debate.

In July 2013, two legislators from towns that had non-profit hospitals considering for-profit acquisition partners attempted to remedy this problem. They sought legislative approval to extend a 2009 law that established medical foundations in the state. A medical foundation is "a mechanism allowing hospitals and certain other health care entities to create nonprofit legal entities to employ physicians or certain other health care providers."[80] At the time, DHN used medical foundations to employee physicians, which was legal because DHN was non-profit.[81] On July 11, 2013, the last night of the session, the two legislators introduced an amendment to an unrelated bill that would allow for-profit entities to open non-profit medical foundations.[82] In this way, for-profit health systems would be able to "spin off" the health-system-owned physician practices to a non-profit entity, meaning that the relationship between the physician organization and the hospital would be one step removed and, most important, legal. Although the bill passed the House and Senate, the governor vetoed the bill, likely due to union pressure.[83]

However, Axiom found a way around this veto. On August 8, 2013, DHN announced it had signed a letter of intent for an acquisition by Axiom *and* Elite University.[84] Elite University would not only bring clinical knowledge, as discussed at the open meeting, but also a way to employ physicians—the university is non-profit and, therefore, permitted to employee physicians through non-profit medical foundations.[85] Axiom indicated that its partnership with Elite University was an interim solution for the problem of state law not allowing a for-profit hospital to employee physicians, since the partnership between Axiom and Elite University could disintegrate at any time. Another way Axiom dealt with the problematic state law was to "outsource" the employment of its full-time hospitalists to an out-of-state, for-profit company, thus avoiding the state law because the physicians would then not be directly employed by a for-profit hospital in the state.[86] The relationship between DHN, Axiom, and Elite University was finalized in March 2014.[87] Likely not a coincidence, in early April 2014 the DHN board of directors approved a definitive agreement of sale to Axiom.[88]

In a second attempt to clear non-profit entities to establish medical foundations, a more permanent solution to what Axiom viewed as the problematic state policy—a bill crafted by Axiom and Elite University lobbyists, which would legalize the practice of for-profit hospitals employing physicians—cleared the state legislature on May 7, 2014.[89] Less than a week later, on May 12, 2014, DHN corporators approved the sale of DHN to Axiom, clearing the way for Axiom to seek regulatory approval for the sale from the state, which was expected to take about a year.[90] The governor signed the bill into law on June 3, 2014.[91]

Unit administrators were aware of the financial constraints the hospital was under and believed that needed equipment and capital investment would be part of the acquisition deal. For example, one administrator told me in a May 2014 interview:

> Sequestration and the budget cuts and everything, you know, [are] looming on the horizon. So, I'm glad to know that we will have that capital reinvestment [due to the acquisition]. There are some things—for example, we've wanted to do a maternal-fetal medicine program here for a long time. But it is a very costly program and we've not been able to support it, and yet that is one of the things that will be part of the new agreement. . . . We need to expand our NICU that . . . we . . . retrofit[ted] into a space that was built when we came here ten years ago and is completely unsuitable for how our NICU has developed. So, knowing that we have a larger partner who's going to help us expand over the next three to five years, that part is very exciting. Certainly, having the linkages with an organization as prestigious as [Elite University] is very exciting. They have a lot to offer us clinically.

The same unit administrator, however, recognized that nurses were fearful of changes: "I think the biggest issue right now is the uncertainty. . . .

I know nurses are afraid they're going to be replaced and . . . lose their benefits, but I don't see that as being a likely outcome."

No doubt she was right about the nurses' perspective. I relay here, too, an interesting observation from my notes in June 2014. At the same time that administrators were embracing the impending changes, nurses and hospital staff were increasingly aware of the hospital's uncertainty, and this caused much anxiety and conflict. For example, Rachel, a soft-spoken, thoughtful nurse, found when she went to put her lunch in the break-room refrigerator that it was full. She walked to the patient kitchen, planning to put her lunch in that refrigerator, which is technically against unit rules but not an uncommon practice. When she arrived at the patient kitchen, one of the kitchen staff was restocking. She asked him if it would be okay for her to put her lunch in the refrigerator. She explained to him that the break-room refrigerator was full. He told her it was fine. However, when he was leaving the unit, he stopped by the front desk and told the charge nurse, Julie, that Rachel should not have put her lunch in the patient refrigerator—it was not appropriate. Then he said something very telling of the uncertainty surrounding the hospital: "When the new company finishes buying the hospital out, they won't tolerate that!" I write about what may seem like a trivial issue because it is indicative of how employees were imagining the changes, however small and insignificant, that would happen with the acquisition.

Changes at DHN continued, despite the impending acquisition, and affected hospital employees directly. In August 2014 Fuller instituted a hiring freeze.[92] Then, in October 2014, Fuller Hospital System laid off around fifty non-union middle-level managers and clerical workers, although Axiom denied that the layoffs were at all affected by the acquisition attempt.[93] Further, in the same month, Fuller froze wages and contributions to the employee pension plan for non-union employees and continued a hiring freeze instituted during the summer months.[94] In addition, unions were asked to revise their contracts to accept similar concessions (i.e., wage freeze and elimination of employer pension plan contributions) for a guarantee of no layoffs for three years, concessions they voted to approve on November 4, 2014.[95]

On December 2, 2014, Axiom's buyout of another hospital in the state was approved by the state Attorney General's Office and the state Department of Public Health's Office of Health Care Access, but with conditions.⁹⁶ These conditions included specifying a dollar value of assets that must be purchased with operating cash and a five-year ban on reducing the level of clinical staff. The conditions were widely speculated to be the template that would be used for the buyout applications of other hospitals in the state, including DHN.⁹⁷ The conditions were too onerous from Axiom's perspective. Axiom notified state officials just over a week later, on December 11, 2014, that it was withdrawing its application to buy DHN (and, in fact, all five of the hospitals it had proposed to buy in the state).⁹⁸

After Axiom: Plan B

DHN had a backup plan to affiliate with another hospital network.⁹⁹ In fact, on January 6, 2015, less than a month after of Axiom's formal withdrawal, DHN sent letters to four for-profit hospital systems and one non-profit hospital system.¹⁰⁰ I was in the hospital during the first week of January when the nurse manager of the OB unit called a staff meeting in which she announced that new suitors were being sought, but that is the only information that was shared. No numbers were given and no information on the systems' location was shared.

She also announced that two new practices would start deliveries at the hospital on March 1, 2015—a practice with obstetricians and midwives and a practice with two midwives, an anticipated addition of two hundred births per year, a 25 percent increase. I suspect that adding these practices was part of plan B. The timing of the announcement is more than coincidental. She told the nurses there would be construction on the unit to add four additional LDRP rooms. When nurses asked if this would be completed by March 1, she said no but that five new postpartum rooms on 3 West would be opened by then, a temporary solution. However, I note here that as of August 2016 construction had not started on the new LDRP rooms. Cynthia, an administrator, told me in an interview in December 2015 that the stalled construction is linked to swift changes in state and national health-care policy. She says:

> It's all on hold until more money comes into this company. . . . The other
> thing that happened . . . in this time period are the . . . changes . . . with

Medicare and Medicaid ... reimbursement, the way they're tying hospital reimbursement to our outcomes. And ... the governor['s] ... projected hospital cuts and everything. ... Things that we thought we had money for ... when you look at a budget ... you think you've got the funds going forward. And then you find out they've been taken away. Well, then other things have to go on hold, and so that's one of the things that's on hold.

DHN received three proposals by March 16, 2015:

One was from a nonprofit system that proposed making a minority investment in DHN, purchasing its home care agency and providing a management agreement for DHN. A second was from a national nonprofit organization that was merging with a [state] nonprofit system and that proposed a member substitution pursuant to which it would become DHN's corporate parent. The third proposal was from Waranoke to acquire all or substantially all of the assets of DHN.[101]

The board of directors evaluated final proposals from the three systems and made the decision to negotiate only with Waranoke. On June 26, 2015, DHN made public that it was focusing solely on Waranoke as an acquirer.[102] Waranoke Health's acquisition application for DHN was due to state regulators by October 5, 2015, but Waranoke was given an extension until November 4, a deadline it met.[103] The acquisition closed on October 1, 2016.

I share here a few more pieces of evidence that shifts in policy are linked to changes at Fuller. First are words from the CEO of DHN. At a public meeting at Marple Hospital, the CEO told the audience:

If the Affordable Care Act is successful, an organization is going to be paid completely differently for caring for the whole patient. ... We recognize that the only way we can be sustainable is if we can get those costs down by 15 percent or 20 percent, and we can't do that any longer.[104]

Notice how the ACA is front and center in the way the executive explains the hospital's crisis. The next piece of evidence comes from the "Statewide Health Care Facilities and Services Plan 2014 Supplement" published by the state's Department of Public Health. The first two key issues identified in this plan concern the impact of the ACA:

- [State's] health care system landscape continues to transform under the Patient Protection and Affordable Care Act (PPACA). The transformation can be seen in the regulatory arena via Certificate of Need (CON) applications received by OHCA [Office of Health Care Access], as providers focus on creating new models of care that bring higher quality at a lower cost, thus delivering greater value in health care.
- Increasingly, [State] hospitals are applying for regulatory approval to become members of umbrella corporate health care systems. These affiliations or mergers may be attributed to several factors, including the economic downturn, health care market competition, PPACA requirements and the need to achieve efficiencies in health care administration and delivery.[105]

Perhaps something even more telling is disclosed later in this report. In the introductory chapter on the current health-care environment, the report reads, "Change in ownership, termination of service, merger of general hospitals and for-profit conversion applications received by OHCA in the past two years have specifically mentioned the PPACA as a reason, in part, for the proposed action." In short, there can be no doubt that what is happening at Fuller Hospital is at least partly due to hospital administrators' response to the ACA.

Fuller Hospital Still in Crisis

Even with a new acquisition deal in the works, it is clear that DHN was still operating in crisis mode as of my final observation in June 2016. Not only were employee salary and benefits concessions still in place, but in July and November 2015 DHN laid off more workers, including thirty-eight managers (one of whom was an administrator in the women's health division) as well as nurses.[106] A DHN spokesperson blamed the layoffs on cuts in Medicaid and Medicare reimbursements and the state's hospital tax. It is the case that the federal government assessed a penalty on the hospital for its readmission rate of Medicare patients being too high. The penalty was a 0.02 percent reduction in Medicare payments from October 1, 2015 through September 30, 2016, and a 1.04 percent reduction from October 1, 2016, through September 30, 2017.[107]

The CEO of DHN publicly announced that the system would cut expenses by 15 to 20 percent. Further, on September 18, 2015, the governor proposed a $64 million reduction in Medicaid funding to hospitals to balance the state budget.[108] In November 2015 DHN announced that to deal with the recent state cuts it would freeze wages for the rest of the fiscal year and continue its suspension of contributions to employee retirement accounts.[109] This announcement came less than two weeks after a local newspaper reported that in 2015 the CEO of DHN was awarded a 41 percent increase in compensation, bringing it to $1.2 million, including $198,000 in incentives and bonus pay, and other administrators received sizable salary increases as well.[110] When I was in the hospital in November 2015 this was a constant source of discussion among the nurses, who strongly believed the compensation to be unfair.

Nurses felt this pinch. My conversations with them revealed that they are looking for employment in other hospitals due to the work environment and uncertainty they now face, and some, even senior nurses, have left for other nursing opportunities. They also recognize the financial impact of not having pay increases or retirement contributions. Ashley discusses her frustration with such a situation:

> ASHLEY: You don't get any money. No raises. They don't match your 401(k). Every time you turn around, they're asking you to come help, but they don't want to pay you the overtime and stuff.
> THERESA: They have to pay overtime, don't they?
> ASHLEY: Well, yeah, in certain circumstances, but they always have excuses for different, you know, there's certain reasons. You've got to meet each criterion for everything. You know, so say you pick up an extra weekend shift. It has to be the full eight hours. If you leave a minute early, they won't give you the bonus rate. Stuff like that.

Crystal is similarly frustrated. She connects the lack of a pay raise to her not feeling like her work is being recognized:

> I think that it's frustrating, because financially, we haven't gotten raises, and I know that's frustrating. It's frustrating to me. . . . I put a lot of hard

hours into here . . . working full-time, and I don't see anything recipro-cated back toward me. . . . I get good remarks . . . on our [patient satis-faction surveys]. I make sure I put the extra effort into our patients, and nothing shows for it. You don't get anything back, and yes, financially, it would be nice to have the little raise here and there, it would. You know, to make a little extra money.

However, Crystal's frustration is not only with lack of financial com-pensation but with the general uncertainty about the security of her job:

And it's stressful because I know they said that . . . it [the Axiom acquisi-tion] fell through, and now they're shopping for new buyers for the hos-pital, and I know they had a contingency plan, but at some point, that's going to run out, too. So, I am concerned about having a job in a couple years . . . because if it doesn't go through, I'm not going to have a job. And it is stressful because then there's going to be a whole bunch of nurses go-ing for the same jobs around the state, and it's going to be a battle. . . . So, it is frustrating that they can't nail this down, and that we are in financial struggles as a hospital, and they're trying to do these little things here and there to try and cut, and they're cutting this, and they're cutting that, and I'm afraid they're going to start cutting the wrong things. And people and patients are going to be the ones who are going to lose, ultimately, because they lose their care.

Crystal is worried about being laid off during the same fiscal year in which executives at the hospital were given large bonuses. In addition to the CEO's raise to $1.2 million in the 2016 fiscal year, the top ten execu-tives collectively were given salaries totaling $5.2 million.[111]

Conclusion

I have argued here that the political-economic environment, including changes introduced by the ACA and by state-level policy changes, has affected Fuller hospital in a way that makes nurses' jobs more difficult. Resource dependence theory predicts that organizational shifts occur in reaction to such tumultuous change, thereby introducing new uncer-tainty into the organization's environment. What is not always clear is how organizations respond to change. There are always hard choices, which typically fall to executives. Thus, one should see the solution to these problems—acquisition by a for-profit hospital—as a choice made by executives. It is important to draw out the political implications of the ACA to the hospital as an organization and, most important, to interactions between real actors (e.g., nurses and patients) within the hospital. This makes visible political economic forces that are often hidden and allows one to see how macro policy decisions actually affect lives.

Conclusion

I think what's going on right now is that the change has been going on for too long. . . . [It has been] a long period of lots and lots of shifting around and reorganization in order to keep this organization alive until we are purchased by a for-profit company. When that happens . . . the expectation is that at some point some more money will be infused into this organization, plus some administrative support. So, right now, we're struggling from the top down because they're just trying to keep the hospital afloat. . . . They've gotten rid of . . . all of the directors, vice presidents and clinical managers . . . and the rest of us have had more and more things piled onto us because there's just less and less support from above. (Cynthia, unit administrator)

Fuller Hospital has been affected by swift and sweeping policy change at the state and national levels, and it is clear that the saga is ongoing. Health-care policy change is, of course, not unique to the time period I cover in this book. However, in the prior chapters I presented a nuanced and in-depth analysis of one hospital's experience with one specific period of policy shifts.

My initial interest in Fuller Hospital was due to the fact that it had some of the best perinatal measures in the state and was seen by doulas, nurses, and midwives as the place to go for a top-notch birth experience. Established by community members, Fuller Hospital had an almost hundred-year-old reputation as an institution that cared for and was deeply embedded in the community. It was one of the first community hospitals in the country to have a dedicated birthing room and was also one of the first U.S. hospitals to offer Lamaze classes.[1] In short, the hospital environment strongly reflected the community's commitment to personalized health care, as evidenced by the local outcry and resistance to the hospital's being purchased by an out-of-state, for-profit corporation.

The Affordable Care Act and state-level cuts in Medicaid funding set in motion new policies and processes that significantly altered the nature of care at Fuller Hospital. In the context of individual community hospitals like Fuller, the ACA has significant consequences, as the policy compels hospitals to increase rules, protocols, and data collection that make patient-oriented nursing very difficult, all while also being expected to meet stepped-up standards of care to maintain current funding levels. These swift changes caused significant upheaval in the daily work of OB nurses and affected their ability to care for patients safely and compassionately.

I have demonstrated throughout this book the different ways nurses support patients, which are often not measured by survey or interview studies. Yet, supporting patients is more and more difficult because nurses at Fuller are now working in an economically struggling hospital under new rules and protocols brought about by the ACA. The hospital has been fined two years in a row for failing to meet ACA-mandated re-admission rates. The fiscal year 2015 (October 1, 2014 through September 30, 2015) penalty was a 0.02 percent reduction in Medicare funding, and the fiscal year 2016 (October 1, 2015 through September 30, 2016) penalty was much higher, 1.04 percent. Fuller Hospital was also penalized for a high infection rate in both 2015 and 2016.[2] Further, Leapfrog gave the hospital a rating of D for patient safety.[3] Nurses have a hard job, one that takes incredible amounts of time, physical and emotional energy, humor, and compassion, all of which is now harder in ways likely not considered by the designers of the ACA.

This is the underbelly of the ACA, especially for small, non-profit, community hospitals. Like Fuller, many community hospitals have been left with no other choice than to merge into a large, for-profit hospital system. These types of acquisitions do not always benefit patient care, and the reason they are pursued by hospitals is that small, community hospitals may have a hard time keeping their doors open without an inflow of capital. Fuller Hospital was already under financial pressures from changes in state-level policies, but the ACA enforced new performance, documentation, and reporting rules of what were termed by the ACA "quality measures." The financial costs of the new rules and procedures proved to be too much for Fuller Hospital. Indeed, the changes brought about a consistent decline in OB patient care and safety. As Jean, an OB nurse at Fuller Hospital, tells me, "If you're not adequately staffed, it becomes unsafe quickly. And we're not in control of who walks in in labor, or who needs a c-section when the emergencies happen, you know?"

My research uses organizational theory to help explain how hospital executives and members of the hospital's board confronted a changing environment in a way predicted by organizational theory—they managed dependencies. They had to deal with funding cuts from the federal and state governments, and internally they restructured employment relationships, compensation, and benefits in order to keep open a financially struggling hospital. Executives of organizations respond to political and economic changes in the environment in ways that promote survival, especially under conditions of uncertainty.[4] However, executive responses also reflect mostly the perspectives and interests of those at the top of the organization, with others (in this case, nurses) being largely left out of the decision making. As Prechel argues in his research, organizational change in response to uncertainty in the environment may introduce irrationalities into the organization.[5] In the case I studied, at least two irrationalities were introduced. First, financial woes were put on the backs of the staff in a way that makes it more difficult for them to do their jobs while at the same time the executives who made the decisions received salary increases and bonuses. Second, and related, separate units and individuals within the hospital were put into competition by the changes and must jockey against each other in ways that are not rational for the stated goals of hospitals—that is, to deliver superior patient care. For example, it is not rational for the OB unit to have to compete with the OR for anesthesiologists or for nurses to compete with one another for basic equipment, such as thermometers, blood pressure cuffs, and telemetry units.

Both patient-oriented and process-oriented nurses are affected by having their salaries and retirement contributions frozen and their health insurance premiums increased. There have been nurse layoffs at the hospital, which, although not experienced yet in the OB unit, still cause uncertainty and anxiety for all nurses at the hospital. Both types of nurses also face the same constraints in terms of aging and missing equipment and handling ever greater numbers of patients.

However, the main argument in this book is that process- and patient-oriented nurses are each affected by these changes in different ways.

Process-oriented nursing is different form patient-oriented nursing in that the primary job responsibility becomes following rules, which includes following protocols and making sure documentation is done correctly. The frustrations of process-oriented nurses lie in their inability to closely follow protocol, which makes them feel vulnerable to claims of malpractice if something goes wrong. A number of these nurses have left their jobs at Fuller, some of them because they felt that birth had become so unsafe at the hospital that a lawsuit was going to happen sooner or later. They did not want to be involved in such a lawsuit, so their solution was to leave.

Patient-oriented nursing provides the care that leads to the best outcome for patient satisfaction, but also for patient health outcomes (e.g., fewer infections due to fewer cervical checks, fewer cesareans because they protect patients from them). However, organizational changes brought about through the ACA affect patient-oriented nursing deeply because they restrict the ability of nurses to provide individualized care to patients. Because individualized compassionate care of patients is the ideal socially constructed role for nurses, changes that affect such care have the potential to significantly alter our basic understanding of nursing in birth and delivery.

Although process- and patient-oriented nurses all contribute toward organizational goals, the implementation of the ACA has shifted the balance so that *all nurses* become more process oriented, with a focus on documentation and the need to care for an increasingly high patient load, leading to a noticeable decline in patient care.

How Can Nurses Advocate for Change?

I cannot make clear enough how much I admire nurses. They are the unsung heroes of patient care. I could not have written this book without the OB nurses of Fuller Hospital welcoming me into their fold. Further, the reason I am writing this book is that it became clear to me in research for my earlier book that nurses are the key to patient care. They are with the patients in the hospital during labor, birth, and the postpartum period. They understand women's bodies and the importance of good patient care. It is with this admiration and respect that I suggest ways nurses might advocate for change.

Nurses should be vocal about any constraints they feel they face in caring for patients. Hospitals increasingly view patients as customers. If those customers know that they may receive less than optimal care at a hospital, they may go elsewhere. Thus, when nurses feel there is danger in hospital practices, like I heard, or that a hospital is no longer a good place at which to give birth, which I also heard, they should let administrators *and* consumers know this. But how are they to do this?

My first suggestion is for nurses to go to the hospital administration with any concerns about safety. Doing so protects the nurse who finds herself involved in providing substandard care due to constraints placed on her by the hospital. Make sure the complaint is documented—like when Evelyn put in "notice" that a stat lab order took too long. Nurses should go to staff, unit, and hospital meetings to voice their concerns and also try to get other nurses to go to those meetings so that they have numbers on their side. It might be easy to ignore or reprimand one nurse who points out problems, but it is not so easy to ignore or reprimand ten or twelve or fifteen nurses, especially in this era of focusing on "patient safety." By making this a patient-safety concern they will not be ignored. Further, nurses should try to get some senior nurses who are secure in their employment to lead the complaints.

A second strategy is to garner public concern so that consumers pressure the hospital for change. I have yet to meet a woman who has given birth or who plans to give birth in the future who is not interested in what OB nurses have to say. When I talk about my research, I am always struck by how much interest and how many questions others have about the nurses. Nurses should talk to more women about their jobs. When asked questions, nurses should answer honestly. They should suggest questions to ask clinicians and hospitals. They should help them to understand that where they give birth is important. A good idea would be for a nurse to give a guest talk to a group like a local chapter of the International Cesarean Awareness Network (ICAN) or the BirthNetwork National to talk about birth and answer any questions that women have.

How Should Women Choose Where to Give Birth?

Given the organizational environment currently affecting hospital OB units, how do women pick a place in which to give birth? Women should do their research about birth choices. I have written about this before, but the information available has gotten decidedly better in the intervening years.[6] It is important to remember that although almost all women in the United States give birth in hospitals, some do give birth at home or in independent birth centers, and these are important options to consider. Although the percentage of women who have out-of-hospital births is low—1.5 percent in 2014—it is increasing.[7] Birth centers have been demonstrated to lead to low levels of obstetrical interventions, including cesareans, as well as low levels of maternal and fetal morbidity.[8] Another study finds that out-of-hospital birth has lower rates of interventions, including cesarean, but also slightly higher fetal death rates, although the fetal death rate is still exceedingly low.[9]

Most women who have a baby in the hospital likely do so by choice, because they were not aware of other options, or because they could not afford an out-of-hospital birth, but sometimes they deliver in hospitals because an out-of-hospital birth is just not an option. There are fewer than four hundred independent birth centers in the United States, although this number is increasing thanks to the ACA's requirement that Medicaid pay birth centers a facility fee.[10] Most home births are attended by certified professional midwives (CPMs). According to Susan Jenkins, an attorney who works on such issues, thirty-three states regulate CPMs, most through licensure. CPMs who practice in one of the seventeen states that do not regulate or authorize CPMs run the risk of being prosecuted for practicing medicine without a license, which often leads to covert types of midwife networks and do not benefit women because transfer to a hospital sometimes become adversarial or, perhaps worse, CPMs may be absent in many or all areas of those states.[11] Further, only two states—Washington and Florida—mandate that state-based health insurance companies cover midwifery care in home births, although some individuals have been successful at convincing health insurers to cover the cost of home birth in other states. In other words, home birth with a trained provider is not available to many women.

For women who decide to give birth in a hospital, important data to compare hospitals is available. First, the Leapfrog group provides comparative data on maternity care on its website, giving individuals access to rates of early elective delivery, cesarean, and episiotomy by hospital.[12] Another source of such data is *Consumer Reports*, which, under the tutelage of Jill Arnold, has accumulated cesarean data on about half of all U.S. hospitals. State Department of Public Health websites may contain hospital data involving birth, although, if they do, *Consumer Reports* likely already has published them. Third, Medicare offers consumers data collected through ACA requirements on the Hospital Compare website (http://medicare.gov/hospitalcompare). Data that women may be interested in involve the hospital-level HCAHPS scores on patient satisfaction and the early delivery statistics. Women should examine data of hospitals in their area to look for the one with the lowest levels of interventions.

What Lies in the Future

Future research should follow up on Fuller Hospital and other hospitals as they change from being a non-profit to a for-profit hospital. There is a substantial literature demonstrating that health outcomes in for-profit hospitals are not as good as those in non-profit hospitals, including research on birth outcomes.[13] It is important to study longitudinally how the change from a not-for-profit to a for-profit hospital affects birth experience and outcomes. Researchers should also keep an eye on health-care consolidation that is proceeding at a quick pace in the United States. What does consolidation mean for individuals and health outcomes? Consolidation is happening across both health insurers as well as hospitals and hospital systems. The latter of these is encouraged by the ACA's focus on Accountable Care Organizations. This is an area ripe for research, and birth outcomes, including mode of delivery and maternal and fetal morbidity and mortality, should be included as outcomes.

I am writing this during a time of uncertainty for the ACA. There is no doubt that future changes are not only possible but likely. President Donald Trump and the congressional Republicans have vowed to repeal the ACA, though with little success, as I am writing in November 2017. It is unclear whether they will succeed, but, if they do, they will likely throw the baby out with the bathwater and, no doubt, will emphasize cutting costs over everything else. The ACA is not perfect, but it also is not a failure. From what I have written, I hope to have demonstrated that consolidation of the health-care industry is a *consequence* of the

ACA. This consolidation does not necessarily benefit the patient, and it undoubtedly makes work life harder for nurses. However, the ACA has brought millions under the health insurance umbrella and improved women's access to reproductive health, a true policy success.

My hope is that Congress will work to keep health-care costs low but with an eye toward how this affects patients as well as hospitals, physicians, and nurses. The interrelationships of the industry must be thought through. Too much distrust in a system breeds problems, and the ACA shows signs of clear distrust of hospitals and health-care providers. Cost of the health-care system cannot be laid on the backs solely of hospitals and health-care providers. For example, one of the reasons our health care costs so much in the United States is that there are problems that run deep in terms of how medical liability works.[14] Reform of the medical liability system is the first place I would suggest to look for cost savings. Reforming this system would lead to fewer unnecessary tests and procedures and more of a focus on evidence-based care rather than on care that *reduces liability*. Solutions to the medical liability system are beyond the scope of this book but have been well researched by other scholars.[15]

Further, it is important to note that women's reproductive health has not been a high priority in our country, and the political assault on women's access to reproductive health care will likely continue under a Trump presidency. For example, women's reproductive and health-care rights have been restricted, especially in the last several years.[16] Women's access to abortion has been seriously constrained, with over 25 percent of abortion restrictions since *Roe v. Wade* enacted between 2010 and 2015.[17] Yet, abortion is not the only area in which women's reproductive rights are constricted. I am currently working on a project involving forced and coerced cesareans and other birth procedures.[18] Some women who refuse a cesarean are forced to have one against their wills, while other women have unconsented episiotomies and are forced or pressured into inductions, labor augmentation, or labor pain relief. Women are also denied access to contraception, midwifery care, and alternative places of birth. This is a full-on attack on women's reproductive health. Perhaps the most egregious indicator of how little our society values women's reproductive health is the high maternal mortality rate in the United States, fourteen per hundred thousand births in 2015, higher than those of Belarus, Croatia, Libya, and Republic of Korea.[19] Something is wrong with how reproductive health care in the United States is delivered, and I fear that the political "solutions" may make matters worse before they get better. We need inclusion of a racially and socioeconomically diverse group of women, mothers, physicians, midwives, nurses, and community members in health-care policy debates and decision making.

ACKNOWLEDGMENTS

I want first to thank all the nurses who let me follow them around for hours on end, armed with my tiny notebook and iPad. They taught me about labor and birth, laughed with me, and shared their work lives with me in a way that helped me to understand. I also thank all the patients and their families who allowed me to watch their care during labor and birth.

Three sociology graduate students—Shelbie Carpenter, Kelly McNamara, and Monica Williams—and two undergraduate students—Amanda Gomez and Faith Duplantis—at Texas A&M University helped in various ways with this project. I am lucky to have the opportunity to work with such smart, talented students. I appreciate the financial support from the Glasscock Humanities Center at Texas A&M University. I was awarded a Glasscock Internal Faculty Fellowship, which was invaluable because it allowed me to focus for the entire fall 2015 semester on writing this book.

Many people have supported this project in various ways—listening, asking questions, suggesting changes—and I have benefited immensely from them: Danielle Bessett, Cathy Kamens, Kelly McNamara, Christine Morton, Harland Prechel, Joan Robinson, Louise Roth, Carrie Lee Smith, and Tim Woods. Of course, any errors that remain are mine alone. I am forever grateful for the confidence Ilene Kalish, my editor at NYU Press, has in my ability to write a good book.

Most important, I thank my family for their never-ending support. My kids, Ben and Allie, cheer me on and make me smile; my husband, Tim, encourages me but, most important, knows when I need a break; and my mom, Susan, reminds me that everything will be okay.

NOTES

INTRODUCTION

1 I give a pseudonym to the hospital, the health systems, and the university that attempted to acquire it.

2 I give pseudonyms to all individuals I write about in the book.

3 Starr, *Remedy and Reaction*.

4 Starr, *Social Transformation of American Medicine*.

5 Ibid.

6 Starr, *Remedy and Reaction*.

7 Uberoi, Finegold, and Gee, "Health Insurance Coverage and the Affordable Care Act."

8 Segal, "Quality/Cost Initiative of PPACA."

9 Radnofsky, "How the ACA May Affect Health Costs."

10 Segal, "Quality/Cost Initiative of PPACA."

11 Morris and McInerney, "Media Representations of Pregnancy and Childbirth."

12 Morris and Schulman, "Race Inequality in Epidural Use and Regional Anesthesia Failure in Labor and Birth"; Morris, Meredith, Schulman, and Morton, "Why Do Low-Risk Women Have C-Sections?"

13 Hamilton et al., "Births."

14 Studying obstetrical nurses is particularly important because they hold a special place in the lives of most women. Although the U.S. birth rate has declined over the past forty years, still 80 percent of U.S. women give birth at some point in their lives. See Livingston and Cohn, "Childless up among All Women." Thus, most women encounter obstetrical nurses at some point during their adult lives.

15 According to the *Merriam-Webster Dictionary*, obstetrics is "a branch of medicine that deals with the birth of children and with the care of women before, during, and after they give birth to children." *Merriam-Webster Dictionary*, s.v. "Obstetrics," n.d., http://www.merriam-webster.com/. Obstetrical nurses are practitioners in this branch of medicine.

16 Hodnett et al., "Continuous Support for Women During Childbirth."

17 Ibid.

18 Ibid.

19 Declercq et al., "Listening to Mothers."

20 Anderson, "Operational Definition of "Support," 17.

21 Ibid.
22 Ibid.
23 Kintz, "Nursing Support in Labor."
24 Roberts, "Factors Influencing Distress from Pain during Labor."
25 Klein et al., "Study of Father and Nurse Support during Labor."
26 Shields, "Nursing Care in Labour and Patient Satisfaction."
27 Ibid.; Kintz, "Nursing Support in Labor."
28 Hamilton et al., "Births."
29 Radin, Harmon, and Hanson, "Nurses' Care During Labor."
30 Ibid.
31 Perrow, "Society of Organizations."
32 Prechel, "Historical Contingency Theory, Policy Paradigm Shifts, and Corporate Malfeasance at the Turn of the 21st Century"; Prechel and Morris, "Effects of Organizational and Political Embeddedness on Financial Malfeasance in the Largest U.S. Corporations"; Prechel et al., "Corporate Diversification Revisited"; Morris, *Cut It Out*; Pfeffer and Salancik, *External Control of Organizations*; Davis and Cobb, "Chapter 2 Resource Dependence Theory."
33 Pfeffer and Salancik, *External Control of Organizations*.
34 Ibid.; Pfeffer, "You're Still the Same."
35 Pfeffer, *Power in Organizations*.
36 Weick, *Social Psychology of Organizing*.
37 Pfeffer and Salancik, *External Control of Organizations*.
38 I know of few studies that ethnographically (i.e., through observational research) examine OB nurses over an extended and continuous period of time. None of the nursing support studies do this, and the few studies of doulas that make such observations look at snapshots to examine the question. This is one of the first works that uses extended observations to study nurses.
39 Ragin, *Comparative Method*, 35.
40 Ibid., 35.
41 Ibid. Many researchers have written case studies of organizations over the years. See, for example, Alvesson, *Management of Knowledge-Intensive Companies*; Barker, *Discipline of Teamwork*; Bosk, *Forgive and Remember*; Bridges, *Reproducing Race*; Burawoy, *Manufacturing Consent*; Collinson, *Managing the Shopfloor*; Delbridge, *Life on the Line in Contemporary Manufacturing*; Down, *Narratives of Enterprise*; Feldman, *Order without Design*; Foner, *Caregiving Dilemma*; Gouldner, *Patterns of Industrial Bureaucracy*; Johnson, *Deinstitutionalising Women*; Kunda, *Engineering Culture*; Latour and Woolgar, *Laboratory Life*; Law, *Organizing Modernity*; Moeran, *Ethnography at Work*; Ogasawara, *Office Ladies and Salaried Men*; Selznick, *TVA and the Grass Roots*; Smith, *Managing in the Corporate Interest*; Watson, *In Search of Management*; Wolcott, *Man in the Principal's Office*; Zabusky, *Launching Europe*; Zald, *Organizational Change*.
42 Kozhimannil, Law, and Virnig, "Cesarean Delivery Rates Vary Tenfold among US Hospitals."

43 Main et al., "Cesarean Deliveries, Outcomes, and Opportunities for Change in California," 9.

44 This importance of place is noted by Tina Rosenberg, who asked in a 2016 New York Times Opinionator blog post:

> You are about to give birth. Pregnancy has gone smoothly. The birth seems as if it will, too. It's one baby, in the right position, full term, and you've never had a cesarean section—in other words, you're at low risk for complications. What's likely to be the biggest influence on whether you will have a C-section?
> A. Your personal wishes.
> B. Your choice of hospital.
> C. Your baby's weight.
> D. Your baby's heart rate in labor.
> E. The progress of your labor.
> The answer is B . . . The rest of the factors do influence the decision. But the hospital determines how these factors are treated.

Rosenberg goes on to detail the very different rates of cesarean by hospital and suggests how, although the other factors in her list are often listed as a cesarean indication, the indications are dealt with differently depending on the hospital. The comments section of the blog is telling. Women and men; mothers and fathers; obstetricians, nurses, and anesthesiologists commented on the post, largely in support of Rosenberg's analysis.

45 Fine and Shulman, "Lies from the Field."

46 Nancy is a pseudonym. I use a different pseudonym for Nancy in the remaining chapters to not share her identity. In this chapter, I talk about Nancy in her specific role on the unit. I do not want to tie this role to the insights I share from her in other chapters. Rather, I discuss the in the remaining chapters the four administrators I interviewed as administrators without specific detail about their administrative roles.

47 In July 2014, I took a one-year leave of absence from Trinity College, where I was a faculty member when I started this study, and began a faculty position at Texas A&M University. Once at Texas A&M, I applied for and received IRB approval from Texas A&M for this study in the fall of 2014. I was employed by both Trinity and Texas A&M between July 2014 and June 2015, and I maintained IRB approval from both places during that time. When I resigned from Trinity College in June 2015, I was no longer required to maintain IRB approval from Trinity College, but I kept my IRB approval up to date with the hospital and Texas A&M University.

CHAPTER 1. WELCOME TO THE OBSTETRIC UNIT

1 Taubenberger and Morens, "1918 Influenza."

2 Lundberg, *Fuller Hospital.*

3 Ibid.

4 Ibid.

5 Fuller Hospital, "History of [Fuller Hospital]," n.d., http://www.echn.org/.

6 O'Brien, "Marple Hospital to Eliminate Childbirth Services."

7 Connecticut Department of Public Health, "Annual Report on the Financial Status of Connecitcut's Short Term Acute Care Hospitals," September 2010, 2015, 2016, http://www.ct.gov/dp.

8 Ibid.

9 Ibid.

10 Michak, "DHN Hospitals Lag on Financial Measures for Third Consecutive Year."

11 Almost all (94 percent) of registered nurses in the United States are women. See Bureau of Labor Statistics, "Labor Force Statistics from the Current Population Survey," February 2017, https://www.bls.gov/. This hospital has exclusively female OB nurses. Thus, when referring to OB nurses, I will use female pronouns.

12 Morris, *Cut It Out.*

13 Another observation that supports the focus on liability occurred a few weeks following a fetal death. The nurses and a doctor were discussing this event, and the doctor told the nurses, "Risk management said that maybe they should have a vaginal birth consent." The family was suing the hospital because the baby died during an attempted vaginal birth.

14 On occasions in which I observed nurses while they cared for patients in rooms near the front desk, I found myself often closing the door to mitigate the noise.

CHAPTER 2. A DAY IN THE LIFE OF AN OBSTETRICAL NURSE

1 A scrub nurse assists in surgery. See Surgery Squad, "C-Section Who Is Involved?" n.d., http://www.surgerysquad.com/. This nurse handles all instruments and hands them to the physician as needed. She also counts all instruments and sponges before and after the surgery to ensure that nothing is left inside the patient. The circulator nurse is involved in all aspects of the surgery. She monitors the patient's vital signs before, during, and after surgery. She also discusses the surgery with the patient before the operation and relays any pertinent information to the anesthesiologist and/or obstetrician. During surgery, the circulator assists the physician and anesthesiologist as needed. Finally, after surgery, the circulator monitors the patient as she comes out of her anesthetic and relays information to the patient's postpartum nurse about any medication or special care the patient will need. In this hospital, the patient's postpartum nurse is the scrub nurse from surgery. Many nurses loathe this role because they say they never get a break. As Julie tells me, "No one ever gives you a lunch break because you're with the patient before, during, and after surgery. You never get a break."

2 Nurses complained that sometimes LPNs from different units were assigned to the overflow unit. What this meant was that only one OB nurse was taking care of five mother-baby pairs, including doing assessments, general care, and discharge. Several complained to me about how hard that was. One nurse told me that when the overflow unit was busy, she asked parents to bring the babies back for manda-

tory newborn screens, such as a hearing screen, because she could not get the tests completed before the patients were ready to be discharged.

3 I found that the keeping of these hours in the book was disputed. I witnessed nurses claiming that their call hours had not been properly recorded. This claim then had to be resolved, which involved several nurses trying to remember who had been on call over the past few months. I also heard a complaint from a nurse who was frustrated that nurses who were preceptors—that is training a new nurse—were not called off. She asked why, if a preceptor had sixteen hours of call and another nurse had twenty hours of call, the nurse with twenty hours of call would be put on call. Another nurse justified the practice, saying that the new nurses needed consistent training. However, it was clear that this practice caused rancor. There had also been a change in the past five years in that the call record reset each year on January 1. Historically, the call record had not reset, which gave huge advantages to those with seniority. Once nurses had been working for several years, they might never be required to go on call because they would have accumulated so many call hours over the years.

4 Secretaries also do tasks that are not specifically their responsibility, like holding newborns or watching siblings while a patient is having an epidural adminis-trated. When secretarial hours were cut, patient care was clearly affected because nurses were taking up the tasks the secretary would normally do and those which she sometimes does even though they are not clearly defined as secretarial or nurse duties.

5 A fetal baseline rate of less than 110 is considered bradycardia, or an abnormally low heart rate. American College of Obstetricians and Gynecologists, "ACOG Practice Bulletin No. 106."

6 I noted something interesting in a January 2014 observation. The medication drawers are labeled with numbers, and when medication is dispensed, the drawer and section it will be in is indicated on the computer screen. I was with Evelyn while she was retrieving ibuprofen for a patient. The computer screen indicates that it is in drawer 5, section 2. But drawer 2 pops out, not drawer 5. I show this to Evelyn, who had not noticed. She told me that pharmacy must have mislabeled the drawers. It occurred to me that this is a substantial patient-safety issue that would be simple to fix. Yet it had been overlooked. One might wonder if over-looking such simple safeguards, such as having the drawers labeled correctly, in favor of the more complicated procedures, such as scanning the patient, nurse, and medication before dispensing any medication, is rational.

7 Nurses are required to document that they have discussed the benefits of breast-feeding with patients, regardless of whether the patient plans to breastfeed. This can be awkward for nurses when the patient has made clear that she does not want to breastfeed.

8 RhoGAM is a shot used to prevent RH disease. The Rh factor makes one's blood "positive" or "negative," so that a person's blood type may be O+ or O−; A+ or A−; B+ or B−; or AB+ or AB−. The Rh factor is inherited. The concern comes

with women who are Rh negative and who become pregnant by a man who is Rh positive. In such a situation, the baby may be either Rh positive or negative. If the baby is Rh positive and the fetus's blood comes in contact with the mother's Rh-negative blood (during pregnancy, labor, or birth), her blood may develop antibodies against the Rh factor, a condition called Rh sensitivity or Rh disease. In future pregnancies these antibodies may destroy fetal red blood cells. Rh sensitivity can be prevented in future pregnancies if the woman receives a shot of Rh immunoglobulin (i.e., RhoGAM) during pregnancy and shortly after birth. See American College of Obstetricians and Gynecologists "Rh Factor."

9 Formed in 2000 by employers and other "large purchasers," the Leapfrog Group has been a leader in collecting data to improve patient safety.

10 Salancik and Pfeffer, "Who Gets Power."

CHAPTER 3. PATIENT-ORIENTED NURSES

1 Pam Smith, in *The Emotional Labour of Nursing Revisited*, discusses nurses as either care oriented or task and hierarchy oriented. However, she does not make this a major distinction in her analysis. I feel it is important to recognize that nurses are not all the same, particularly in terms of how they care for patients, and thus this distinction is central to my analysis.

2 American College of Obstetricians and Gynecologists et al., "Safe Prevention of the Primary Cesarean Delivery"; Leveno, Nelson, and McIntire, "Second-Stage Labor"; Spong et al., "Preventing the First Cesarean Delivery."

3 Gimovsky and Berghella, "Randomized Controlled Trial of Prolonged Second Stage."

4 I found it difficult to find an exact definition of a medical-surgical unit to furnish here. The University of California at Davis has the easiest and clearest definition I found of what such a unit does. They define their medical-surgical unit as one that "manages acute medical surgical patients with a wide range of diagnoses and care needs" See UC Davis Medical Center, "Nursing," n.d., http://www.ucdmc. ucdavis.edu/.

5 Clark et al., "Neonatal and Maternal Outcomes Associated with Elective Term Delivery."

6 Some physicians who deliver at this hospital make it a practice to begin inductions at night.

7 In my observations, this physician often discussed liability risks. Liability seemed to be always on her mind.

8 I write "may be more likely" because the evidence is not clear. L. M. Harper and colleagues, in "Association of Induction of Labor and Uterine Rupture in Women Attempting Vaginal Birth after Cesarean: A Survival Analysis," found that uterine rupture risk is not more likely for women with a previous cesarean who are induced compared to women with a previous cesarean who begin labor spontaneously. Further, a Cochrane review on this topic concludes that there is insufficient evidence to suggest whether labor induction has more risks than repeat cesar-

ean or to evaluate which induction agent has the least risk. See also Dodd et al., "Elective Repeat Caesarean Section versus Induction of Labour for Women with a Previous Caesarean Birth"; Jozwiak and Dodd, "Methods of Term Labour Induction for Women with a Previous Caesarean Section."

9 Morris, *Cut It Out*; Alfirevic, Devane, and Gyte, "Continuous Cardiotocography (CTG) as a Form of Electronic Fetal Monitoring (EFM) for Fetal Assessment during Labor."

10 Ibid.

11 AWHONN, *Guidelines for Professional Registered Nurse Staffing for Perinatal Units*.

12 In general, I tried not to answer when asked questions about what was happing in the OB unit because I felt it was outside my role and also because I did not want to provide incorrect information. However, in this case, I also sensed the pressure the unit and its nurses were under and felt it almost unethical to withhold information I knew to be correct.

13 Straight cath refers to intermittent catheterization. The urine is drained from the bladder, and the catheter is taken out.

14 Preeclampsia Foundation, "Signs and Symptoms," n.d., http://www.preeclampsia.org/.

15 I was in the unit the day before, and a baby was screaming in the NICU. The screams were piercing and persistent, and could be heard throughout the unit. There is no doubt that the charge nurse and, quite frankly, everyone on the unit—patient, nurse, doctor, staff, sociology researcher—heard the baby's screams.

16 Mayo Clinic, "Diseases and Conditions: Preeclampsia—Tests and Diagnosis," n.d., http://www.mayoclinic.org/.

17 I do not go with them because I have not consented that patient, and it is not ethnical to consent a patient in this stage of labor.

18 Recall Evelyn's dismay when a resident placed Cytotec vaginally in a patient and her direct conversation with the midwife supervising the resident about how that should never happen again.

19 Placental abruption is a rare risk of ECV. See Grootscholten et al., "External Cephalic Version-Related Risks."

20 The physician, although not new by any means, asked another physician with what dose to medicate the patient in order to bring her blood pressure down. I wrote in my notes: "That just totally made me feel insecure for that patient because she [the physician] seemed not to know [the medication to use or the dose]. She didn't seem that concerned about it either."

21 When I ask Lori to explain why a fetal elevated heart rate is an indication of maternal fever, she tells me that when anyone has a fever his or her heart rate increases. Thus, a fetus's heart rate increases, too, if the maternal temperature goes up. See Sweha, Hacker, and Nuovo, "Interpretation of the Electronic Fetal Heart Rate During Labor."

22 Nurses use what Arlie Russell Hochschild in *The Managed Heart* refers to as emotional labor in their work. OB nurses are expected to display certain emotions by

both the OB managers and the patients. For example, OB nurses are expected to be pleasant, nurturing, and intimately interested in their patients, and this is true regardless of the type of day they are having or how difficult a certain patient may be. Emotional labor is hard work, as documented by Hochschild in her study of flight attendants, and it takes a toll on nurses. For instance, Hochschild suggests that when moods or emotions become a product that must be used in daily work, it belongs more to the organization than it does the individual.

23 American College of Obstetricians and Gynecologists, "ACOG Issues Guidelines on Fetal Macrosomia."

24 Thank you to family physician (and friend) Cathy Kamens for explaining to me the use of scissors in labor and birth.

25 O'Connor et al., "Pacifiers and Breastfeeding."

26 In the end, no one received a bonus because the union told the hospital that if one unit is giving a signing bonus that all units must give a signing bonus. The unit then rescinded the offer of a bonus.

27 The condition necessitating the induction is rare, and I do not mention it here so as not to potentially identify the patient.

28 American College of Obstetricians and Gynecologists. "ACOG Practice Bulletin No. 106."

CHAPTER 4. PROCESS-ORIENTED NURSES

1 Martin, "Giving Birth Like a Girl."

2 Centers for Disease Control and Prevention, "2015 Natality Public Use File Documentation," last modified July 25, 2016, http://www.cdc.gov/.

3 Algert et al., "Labor before a Primary Cesarean Delivery."

4 This perspective is what Arlie Russell Hochschild in *The Managed Heart* refers to as deep acting because the employee's emotions are aligned with the needs of the organization. Also, one of the core issues organizational theory deals with is how organizations attempt to align employee behavior with organizational goals. See Jaffee, *Organization Theory*.

5 Rh sensitization can also occur if the women has an amniocentesis, chronic villus sampling, bleeding during pregnancy, external cephalic version (to manually reposition a fetus from breech to head-down presentation before labor begins), or blunt trauma to the abdomen during pregnancy (American College of Obstetricians and Gynecologists, "Rh Factor").

6 American College of Obstetricians and Gynecologists, "Approaches to Limit Interventions during Labor and Birth."

7 Bretelle, Le Du, and Foulhy, "Modality of Fetal Heart Monitoring during Labor (Continuous or Intermittent), Telemetry, and Central Fetal Monitoring."

8 Rostow and Bulger, *Medical Professional Liability and the Delivery of Obstetrical Care.*

9 Keating, "Hospitals Go Head-to-Head with Malloy."

10 Ohlsson and Shah, "Intrapartum Antibiotics for Known Maternal Group B Streptococcal Colonization."

11 It is important to recognize that each time the cervix is checked, the risk of infection goes up because a foreign body (in the form of fingers of the nurse or physician) is introduced into the vagina.

12 Although it is still a common belief that administration of an epidural before a woman's cervix is dilated to four or five centimeters may make a cesarean more likely, this belief has been challenged by the latest Cochrane report, which finds no correlation between early or late initiation of epidural and mode of delivery. Ban Leong Sng and colleagues conclude, "For first time mothers in labour who request epidurals for pain relief, it would appear that the time to initiate epidural analgesia is dependent upon women's requests." This might be particularly the case when the women are not encouraged to walk or use some other form of pain relief, such as rocking on a birth ball. See Ban Leong Sng et al., "Early versus Late Initiation of Epidural Analgesia for Labour," 2.

13 The car seat test is designed to ensure that babies under thirty-seven weeks' gestation and/or under 2,500 grams (about 5.5 pounds) have adequate oxygen levels and normal breathing when they are in car seats. See American Academy of Pediatrics: Committe on Injury and Poison Prevention and Committee on Fetus and Newborn, "Safe Transportation of Premature and Low Birth Weight Infants." Babies must be monitored for ninety minutes. This is a significant drain on a nurse's time because she is not relieved of patient duties when she conducts this test. Babies also often scream during the test, making it emotionally taxing to administer.

14 Nurses would sometimes call the desk before a mandatory call time was coming up to see if they would need to come in. Liv likely had signed up for call from 11:00 to 3:00 and was checking to see if she needed to come in at 11:00.

15 Johns Hopkins Medicine, "Non-stress Test (NST)," n.d., http://www.hopkinsmedicine.org/.

16 Stevens et al., "Sucrose for Analgesia in Newborn Infants Undergoing Painful Procedures."

17 Recall that all newborns wear a security bracelet that causes an alarm to sound if the tag gets too close to a door or if it is removed.

18 Alfirevic, Devane, and Gyte, "Continuous Cardiotocography (CTG) as a Form of Electronic Fetal Monitoring (EFM) for Fetal Assessment during Labor."

CHAPTER 5. HEALTH-CARE POLICY CHANGES AND
ORGANIZATIONAL CRISIS

1 U.S. Department of Health and Human Services, "2011 Report to Congress."

2 Blumenthal, Abrams, and Nuzum, "Affordable Care Act at 5 Years," 2542.

3 Starr, *Remedy and Reaction.*

4 Ibid.

5 Ibid., 205.
6 Stefan et al., "Hospital Performance Measures and 30-Day Readmission Rates"; Barnett, Hsu, and McWilliams, "Patient Characteristics and Differences in Hospital Readmission Rates"; Calvillo-King et al., "Impact of Social Factors on Risk of Readmission or Mortality in Pneumonia and Heart Failure"; Damiani et al., "Influence of Socioeconomic Factors on Hospital Readmissions for Heart Failure and Acute Myocardial Infarction in Patients 65 Years and Older"; Kurtz et al., "Hospital, Patient, and Clinical Factors Influence 30- and 90-Day Readmission after Primary Total Hip Arthroplasty"; Kurtz et al., "Which Clinical and Patient Factors Influence the National Economic Burden of Hospital Readmissions after Total Joint Arthroplasty?"
7 Sommer, "Gripes about Obamacare Aside, Health Insurers Are in a Profit Spiral."
8 Blumenthal, Abrams, and Nuzum, "Affordable Care Act at 5 Years."
9 Kahn et al., "Assessing Medicare's Hospital Pay-for-Performance Programs and Whether They Are Achieving Their Goals."
10 Blumenthal, Abrams, and Nuzum, "Affordable Care Act at 5 Years."
11 Berenson, Paulus, and Kalman, "Medicare's Readmissions-Reduction Program."
12 Joynt and Jha, "Thirty-Day Readmissions"; Feemster and Au, "Penalizing Hospitals for Chronic Obstructive Pulmonary Disease Readmissions."
13 Blumenthal, Abrams, and Nuzum, "Affordable Care Act at 5 Years."
14 Chedekel, "18 State Hospitals Penalized for High Infection Rates."
15 Blumenthal, Abrams, and Nuzum, "Affordable Care Act at 5 Years."
16 Wolosin, Ayala, and Fulton, "Nursing Care, Inpatient Satisfaction, and Value-Based Purchasing."
17 Blumenthal, Abrams, and Nuzum, "Affordable Care Act at 5 Years."
18 Wolosin, Ayala, and Fulton, "Nursing Care, Inpatient Satisfaction, and Value-Based Purchasing"; Kavanagh et al., "Moving Healthcare Quality Forward with Nursing-Sensitive Value-Based Purchasing"; Kurtzman, Dawson, and Johnson, "Current State of Nursing Performance Measurement, Public Reporting, and Value-Based Purchasing."
19 Pfeffer and Salancik, *External Control of Organizations.*
20 Werner and Dudley, "Medicare's New Hospital Value-Based Purchasing Program Is Likely to Have Only a Small Impact on Hospital Payments."
21 Blumenthal, Abrams, and Nuzum, "Affordable Care Act at 5 Years."
22 U.S. Legal, "Episode of Care (Health Care) Law and Legal Definition," n.d., http://definitions.uslegal.com/.
23 Centers for Medicare and Medicaid Services, "Bundled Payments for Care Improvement Initiative Fact Sheet," January 30, 2014, http://www.cms.gov/; Delbanco, "Payment Reform Landscape."
24 Shortell, Casalino, and Fisher, "How the Center for Medicare and Medicaid Innovation Should Test Accountable Care Organizations."
25 Burke, "Accountable Care Organizations."
26 Blumenthal, Abrams, and Nuzum, "Affordable Care Act at 5 Years," 2454.

27 McWilliams and Song, "Implications for ACOs of Variations in Spending Growth."

28 Gold, "Accountable Care Organizations, Explained."

29 Phipps-Taylor and the West Coast Harkness Policy Forum, "Getting to the ACO Tipping Point"; Muhlestein, "Growth and Dispersion of Accountable Care Organizations in 2015"; Fisher et al., "Framework for Evaluating the Formation, Implementation, and Performance of Accountable Care Organizations."

30 Phipps-Taylor and the West Coast Harkness Policy Forum, "Getting to the ACO Tipping Point"; Miller, "Inside Health-Reform Savings"; McWilliams et al., "Performance Differences in Year 1 of Pioneer Accountable Care Organizations."

31 Muhlestein and McClellan, "Accountable Care Organizations in 2016."

32 Ibid.

33 Muhlestein, "Growth and Dispersion of Accountable Care Organizations in 2015."

34 For a good summary of the different types of ACOs, see ibid.

35 Goldsmith, "Accountable Care Organizations," 32.

36 Horwitz, "ACA's Hospital Tax-Exemption Rules and the Practice of Medicine"; Horwitz, "Does Nonprofit Ownership Matter?"; Madoff, "How the Government Gives."

37 Horwitz, "ACA's Hospital Tax-Exemption Rules and the Practice of Medicine."

38 Ibid.

39 Ibid.; Internal Revenue Service, "New Requirements for 501(c)(3) Hospitals under the Affordable Care Act," n.d., http://www.irs.gov/.

40 Ibid.

41 Folkemer et al., "Hospital Community Benefits after the ACA."

42 Becker, Cerny, and Timmerman, "Hospital Tax-Exempt Status," 3.

43 Rudowitz, "Issue Brief."

44 Centers for Medicare and Medicaid Services, "Disproportionate Share Hospital," last modified August 2, 2017, http://www.cms.gov/.

45 Associated Press, "Will Safety Net Hospitals Survive Health Reform?"

46 Rosenbaum, "Tax-Exempt Status For Nonprofit Hospitals under ACA"; Rosenbaum, "Additional Requirements for Charitable Hospitals."

47 Internal Revenue Service, "New Requirements for 501(c)(3) Hospitals under the Affordable Care Act," last modified August 17, 2017, http://irs.gov/.

48 Horwitz, "ACA's Hospital Tax-Exemption Rules and the Practice of Medicine."

49 American Hospital Association, "Ernst & Young Schedule H Benchmark Report for the American Hospital Association Tax Years 2009 and 2010," n.d., http://www.aha.org/.

50 Ibid.

51 Howley, "Obamacare Installs New Scrutiny, Fines for Charitable Hospitals That Treat Uninsured People."

52 Gold, "Mergers of For-Profit, Non-Profit Hospitals," 1.

53 Ibid.; see also Centers for Disease Control, "Health, United States," various years, available at https://www.cdc.gov/.

54 Weisman, "Equity Firm Set to Buy Caritas"; Mrozinski, "Purchase of Mercy Hospital Could Return Nearly $1 Million to Local Tax Rolls."

55 Blumenthal, Abrams, and Nuzum, "Affordable Care Act at 5 Years," 2456.

56 Casalino and Bishop, "Symbol of Health System Transformation?"

57 Blumenthal, Abrams, and Nuzum, "Affordable Care Act at 5 Years."

58 Goodman, "Six Problems with the ACA That Aren't Going Away."

59 Creswell and Abelson, "New Laws and Rising Costs Create a Surge of Supersizing Hospitals."

60 Ibid.

61 Ibid.

62 Hartocollis, "2 Hospital Networks Agree to Merge, Raising Specter of Costlier Care."

63 Vogt and Town, "How Has Hospital Consolidation Affected the Price and Quality of Hospital Care?"

64 Goldsmith, "Accountable Care Organizations".

65 Richman and Schulman, "Cautious Path Forward on Accountable Care Organizations."; Crosson and Combes, "We'll Need a Bigger Boat"; Kocher and Sahni, "Hospitals' Race to Employ Physicians."

66 Crosson and Combes, "We'll Need a Bigger Boat"; Kocher and Sahni, "Hospitals' Race to Employ Physicians."

67 Devers and Berenson, "Can Accountable Care Organizations Improve the Value of Health Care by Solving the Cost and Quality Quandaries?" 1.

68 Ibid., 3.

69 State of Connecticut and Department of Revenue Services, "2011 Legislation Imposing the Hospital Net Patient Revenue Tax Act," November 8, 2011, http://www.ct.gov/.

70 Buck, "Hospitals Say Malloy's Proposed Tax Will Harm Their Financial Health."

71 Prince, "Battle Emerging over Proposed Tax on Nonprofit Hospitals"; Vigdor, "Malloy Stays the Course with Controversial Plan to Tax Hospitals"; Becker, "CT's Hospital Spending and Taxes, Explained"; Phaneuf and Pazniokas, "Lembo Joins Dissent over Malloy's Emergency Budget Cuts"; "Fleecing Hospitals to Fix State Budget"; Connecticut Department of Public Health, "Annual Report on the Financial Status of Connecticut's Short Term Acute Care Hospitals."

72 Becker, "CT's Hospital Spending and Taxes, Explained."

73 Directional Health Network, "Waranoke to Acquire Both Fuller and Marple as Part of Acquisition of DHN," docket no. 15-32016-486, merger application provided by Connecticut Department of Public Health, 2015, available at http://wwww.ct.gov/dph.

74 Ibid.

75 Ibid.

76 Prechel and Morris, "Effects of Organizational and Political Embeddedness on Financial Malfeasance in the Largest U.S. Corporations."

77 Directional Health Network, "Waranoke to Acquire Both Fuller and Marple as Part of Acquisition of DHN."

78 Ibid.

79 Ibid.

80 James Orlando, "Medical Foundations," June 25, 2013, http://www.cga.ct.gov/.

81 Jacovino, "Axiom's Way Eased."

82 Orlando, "Medical Foundations"; Jacovino, "Bill Vetoed That Would Have Allowed More for Profits to Buy Hospitals."

83 Jacovino, "Malloy Signs Bill Aiding DHN Sale"; Jacovino, "Bill Vetoed That Would Have Allowed More for Profits to Buy Hospitals."

84 Jacovino, "DHN Picks Suitor."

85 Michak, "Axiom's Way around Governors's Veto Is Elite University."

86 Michak, "Doctor Is Out—West."

87 Michak, "DHN Hospitalist Company Used by Axiom"

88 Michak and Kennedy, "Approved but Not OK."

89 Jacovino, "Axiom's Way Eased."

90 Stankiewicz, "DHN System Corporators OK Sale."

91 Jacovino, "Malloy Signs Bill Aiding DHN Sale."

92 Michak, "DHN Faces 'Extraordinary Challenges.'"

93 Soper, "Directional Hospital System Hospital System Laying Off Managers while Negotiating Nurses Contract"; Michak, "Axiom Denies Layoff Role"; Michak, "DHN Faces 'Extraordinary Challenges.'"

94 Michak, "DHN Faces 'Extraordinary Challenges.'"

95 Ibid.; Michak, "Unionized DHN Employees Trade Contract Concessions for Job Security."

96 Sturdevant, "State Regulators Aprpove Joint Venutre of Axiom, Waterbury Hospital, with Conditions."

97 Ibid.; Pazniokas, "Battle Lines Drawn over Conditions on Waterbury Hospital Deal."

98 Michak, "Axiom Calls It Quits"; Pazniokas, "Axiom Ends Bid to Acquire Connecticut Hospitals." The story does not end there. DHN executives pled with the governor to persuade Axiom to come back to the table while at the same time keeping the option open to merge with other health systems. Pazniokas, "Axiom Ends Bid to Acquire Connecticut Hospitals." State senators persuaded Axiom to visit the state to personally talk with them in early January 2015. Michak and Savino, "DHN Pleads for Help." Shortly after Axiom's scheduled meeting with senators was reported in local newspapers, the governor sent a letter to Axiom requesting that they speak to him about reconsidering their decision, although when Axiom received the letter they declined to comment to local press. Haar, "Hope for a Revival of Axiom Hospital Deal." Newspapers reported that Axiom's president and CEO sent a letter to the governor, dated January 19, 2015, indicating that Axiom would speak with the governor's chief of staff, but that in order for the

acquisition bid to proceed the state would have to agree to predetermined conditions that would apply to all acquisitions of hospitals in the state (each acquisition that Axiom wanted was to have gone through separate state regulatory approval). Haar, "Malloy to Axiom"; Sturdevant, "Axiom Declines to Comment on Malloy Letter." However, on February 4, 2015, Axiom and the governor issued a joint statement that negotiations had ended and that Axiom would not be acquiring any hospitals in the state. Michak, "Axiom Gives Malloy Terms to Revive Hospital Buyout Plans"; Sturdevant, "Axiom CEO Skewers Regulatory Environmnet, but Is Open to a Deal."

 99 Michak, "Axiom Calls It Quits,"; Sturdevant, "Axiom Declines to Comment on Malloy Letter."
100 Directional Health Network, "Waranoke to Acquire Both Fuller and Marple as Part of Acquisition of DHN."
101 Ibid., 40.
102 Michak, "DHN's New Suitor Owned by a Buyout Firm."
103 Michak, "Deadline Extended for DHN and Scout."
104 Michak and Kennedy, "Approved but Not OK," 3.
105 Connecticut Department of Public Health, "Statewide Health Care Facilities and Services Plan."
106 Michak, "DHN Sheds More Jobs."
107 Ibid.
108 Phaneuf and Pazniokas, "Lembo Joins Dissent over Malloy's Emergency Budget Cuts."
109 Michak, "DHN Blames State Cuts for Wage Freeze, Stops Retirement Account Contributions."
110 Michak, "Execs Loot DHN on Eve of Sale."
111 Ibid.

CONCLUSION

 1 Lundberg, *Fuller Hospital*.
 2 Chedekel, "18 State Hospitals Penalized for High Infection Rates."
 3 Soper, "Safety Grade Slips for Hospitals."
 4 Pfeffer and Salancik, *External Control of Organizations*; Prechel and Morris, "Effects of Organizational and Political Embeddedness on Financial Malfeasance in the Largest U.S. Corporations"; Prechel, "Irrationality and Contradiction in Organizational Change."
 5 Prechel, "Irrationality and Contradiction in Organizational Change."
 6 Morris, *Cut It Out*.
 7 MacDorman and Declercq, "Trends in Characteristics in United States Out-of-Hospital Births."
 8 Stapleton, Osborne, and Illuzzi, "Outcomes of Care in Birth Centers."
 9 Snowden et al., "Planned Out-of-Hospital Birth and Birth Outcomes."

10 Galewitz, "Not a Hospital, Not a Home Birth." This change in legislation has been credited with their spread because, with Medicaid being the insurer for half of all U.S. births, birth centers are now more economically feasible.

11 States that do not regulate or authorize CPMs as of October 2017 are Connecticut, Hawaii, Illinois, Iowa, Kansas, Kentucky, Massachusetts, Mississippi, Nebraska, Nevada, North Carolina, North Dakota, Ohio, Oklahoma, Pennsylvania, Vermont, and West Virginia.

12 See the Leapfrog Group website at http://www.leapfroggroup.org/.

13 Morris, McNamara, and Morton, "Hospital Ownership Status and Cesareans in the United States"; "Devereaux et al., "Comparison of Mortality between Private For-Profit and Private Not-for-Profit Hemodialysis Centers"; Devereaux et al., "Systematic Review and Meta-Analysis of Studies Comparing Mortality Rates of Private For-Profit and Private Not-for-Profit Hospitals."

14 Mello, Studdert, and Kachalia, "Medical Liability Climate and Prospects for Reform."

15 Ibid.; Mello, Kachalia, and Studdert, "Administrative Compensation for Medical Injuries"; Barringer et al., "Administrative Compensation of Medical Injuries"; Mello et al., "'Health Courts' and Accountability for Patient Safety."

16 Denbow, *Governed through Choice.*

17 Guttmacher Institute, "Last Five Years Account for More Than One-Quarter of All Abortion Restrictions Enacted since Roe," January 13, 2016, http://www.guttmacher.org/.

18 Morris and Robinson, "Forced and Coerced Cesarean Sections."

19 World Health Organization, "Trends in Maternal Mortality, 1990–2015," n.d., http://www.who.int/.

BIBLIOGRAPHY

Alfirevic, Zarko, Declan Devane, and Gillian ML Gyte. "Continuous Cardioto-cography (CTG) as a Form of Electronic Fetal Monitoring (EFM) for Fetal Assessment during Labor." *Cochrane Database of Systematic Reviews* 5 (2013): CD006066.

Algert, C. S., J. M. Morris, J. M. Simpson, J. B. Ford, and C. L. Roberts. "Labor before a Primary Cesarean Delivery: Reduced Risk of Uterine Rupture in a Subsequent Trial of Labor for Vaginal Birth after Cesarean." *Obstetrics and Gynecology* 112, no. 5 (November 2008): 1061–66.

Alvesson, Mats. *Management of Knowledge-Intensive Companies*. Berlin: Walter de Gruyter, 1995.

American Academy of Pediatrics: Committee on Injury and Poison Prevention and Committee on Fetus and Newborn. "Safe Transportation of Premature and Low Birth Weight Infants." *Pediatrics* 97, no. 5 (1996): 758–60.

American College of Obstetricians and Gynecologists. "ACOG Issues Guidelines on Fetal Macrosomia." *American Family Physician* 64, no. 1 (2001): 169–70.

———. "ACOG Practice Bulletin No. 106: Intrapartum Fetal Heart Rate Monitoring: Nomenclature, Interpretation, and General Management Principles." *Obstetrics and Gynecology* 114, no. 1 (July 2009): 192–202.

———. "Approaches to Limit Intervention During Labor and Birth." *ACOG Committee Bulletin* 687 (February 2017). https://www.acog.org/.

———. "The Rh Factor: How It Can Affect Your Pregnancy." *ACOG FAQ027* (September 2013). https://www.acog.org/.

American College of Obstetricians and Gynecologists, Society for Maternal-Fetal Medicine, A. B. Caughey, A. G. Cahill, J. M. Guise, and D. J. Rouse. "Safe Prevention of the Primary Cesarean Delivery." *American Journal of Obstetrics and Gynecology* 210, no. 3 (March 2014): 179–93.

Anderson, Claudia. "Operational Definition of 'Support.'" *Journal of Obstetric, Gynecologic, and Neonatal Nursing* 5, no. 1 (1976): 17–18.

Associated Press. "Will Safety Net Hospitals Survive Health Reform?" *NBC News*, September 8, 2009.

AWHONN. *Guidelines for Professional Registered Nurse Staffing for Perinatal Units*. Washington, DC: AWHONN, 2010.

Barker, James R. *The Discipline of Teamwork: Participation and Concertive Control*. Thousand Oaks, CA: Sage, 1999.

Barnett, M. L., J. Hsu, and J. McWilliams. "Patient Characteristics and Differences in Hospital Readmission Rates." *JAMA Internal Medicine* 175, no. 11 (2015): 1803–12.

Barringer, P. J., D. M. Studdert, A. B. Kachalia, and M. M. Mello. "Administrative Compensation of Medical Injuries: A Hardy Perennial Blooms Again." *Journal of Health Politics, Policy, and Law* 33, no. 4 (August 2008): 725–60.

Becker, Arielle Levin. "CT's Hospital Spending and Taxes, Explained." *Connecticut Mirror*, October 19, 2015.

Becker, Scott, Milton Cerny, and Anna Timmerman. "Hospital Tax-Exempt Status: Considerations Regarding Maintaining Exempt Status." *Becker's Hospital Review*, May 10, 2011.

Berenson, Robert A., Ronald A. Paulus, and Noah S. Kalman. "Medicare's Readmissions-Reduction Program—a Positive Alternative." *New England Journal of Medicine* 366, no. 15 (2012): 1364–66.

Blumenthal, David, Melinda Abrams, and Rachel Nuzum. "The Affordable Care Act at 5 Years." *New England Journal of Medicine* 372, no. 25 (2015): 2451–58.

Bosk, Charles L. *Forgive and Remember: Managing Medical Failure*. Chicago: University of Chicago Press, 1979.

Bretelle, F., R. Le Du, and C. Foulhy. "Modality of Fetal Heart Monitoring during Labor (Continuous or Intermittent), Telemetry, and Central Fetal Monitoring." *Journal of Gynecology Obstetrics and Human Reproduction* 37, no. S1 (February 2008): S23–33.

Bridges, Khiara M. *Reproducing Race: An Ethnography of Pregnancy as a Site of Racialization*. Berkeley: University of California Press, 2011.

Buck, Rinker. "Hospitals Say Malloy's Proposed Tax Will Harm Their Financial Health." *Hartford Courant*, April 21, 2011.

Burawoy, Michael. *Manufacturing Consent: Changes in the Labor Process under Monopoly Capitalism*. Chicago: University of Chicago Press, 1979.

Burke, Taylor. "Accountable Care Organizations." *Public Health Reports* 126, no. 6 (November/December 2011): 875–78.

Calvillo-King, L., D. Arnold, K. J. Eubank, M. Lo, P. Yunyongying, H. Stieglitz, and E. A. Halm. "Impact of Social Factors on Risk of Readmission or Mortality in Pneumonia and Heart Failure: Systematic Review." *Journal of General Internal Medicine* 28, no. 2 (February 2013): 269–82.

Casalino, Lawrence P., and Tara F. Bishop. "Symbol of Health System Transformation? Assessing the CMS Innovation Center." *New England Journal of Medicine* 372, no. 21 (2015): 1984–85.

Chedekel, Lisa. "18 State Hospitals Penalized for High Infection Rates." *Connecticut Mirror*, December 21, 2015.

Clark, S. L., D. D. Miller, M. A. Belfort, G. A. Dildy, D. K. Frye, and J. A. Meyers. "Neonatal and Maternal Outcomes Associated with Elective Term Delivery." *American Journal of Obstetrics and Gynecology* 200, no. 2 (February 2009): 156.e1–4.

Collinson, David L. *Managing the Shopfloor: Subjectivity, Masculinity and Workplace Culture*. Berlin: Walter de Gruyter, 1992.

Connecticut Department of Public Health. "Statewide Health Care Facilities and Services Plan, 2014 Supplement," February 15, 2015. http://www.ct.gov/dph.

Creswell, Julie, and Reed Abelson. "New Laws and Rising Costs Create a Surge of Supersizing Hospitals." *New York Times*, August 12, 2013.

Crosson, Francis J., and John Combes. "We'll Need a Bigger Boat: Reimagining the Hospital-Physician Partnership." *Health Affairs Blog* (blog), April 17, 2014. http://healthaffairs.org/blog/.

Damiani, G., E. Salvatori, G. Silvestrini, I. Ivanova, L. Bojovic, L. Iodice, and W. Ricciardi. "Influence of Socioeconomic Factors on Hospital Readmissions for Heart Failure and Acute Myocardial Infarction in Patients 65 Years and Older: Evidence from a Systematic Review." *Clinical Interventions in Aging* 10 (2015): 237–45.

Davis, Gerald, and J. Adam Cobb. "Chapter 2 Resource Dependence Theory: Past and Future: Stanford's Organization Theory Renaissance, 1970–2000." *Research in the Sociology of Organizations* 28, no. 1 (2010): 21–42.

Declercq, Eugene R., Carol Sakala, Maureen P. Corry, Sandra Applebaum, and Ariel Herrlich. *Listening to Mothers III: Pregnancy and Birth*, edited by Childbirth Connection. New York: Childbirth Connection, 2013.

Delbanco, Suzanne. "The Payment Reform Landscape: Bundled Payment." *Health Affairs Blog* (blog), July 2, 2014. http://healthaffairs.org/blog/.

Delbridge, Rick. *Life on the Line in Contemporary Manufacturing: The Workplace Experience of Lean Production and the "Japanese" Model.* Oxford, UK: Oxford University Press, 2003.

Denbow, Jennifer M. *Governed through Choice: Autonomy, Technology, and the Politics of Reproduction.* New York: New York University Press, 2015.

Devereaux, P. J., P. T. Choi, C. Lacchetti, B. Weaver, H. J. Schunemann, T. Haines, J. N. Lavis, et al. "A Systematic Review and Meta-Analysis of Studies Comparing Mortality Rates of Private For-Profit and Private Not-for-Profit Hospitals." *CMAJ* 166, no. 11 (May 2002): 1399–1406.

Devereaux, P. J., H. J. Schunemann, N. Ravindran, M. Bhandari, A. X. Garg, P. T. Choi, B. J. Grant, et al. "Comparison of Mortality between Private For-Profit and Private Not-for-Profit Hemodialysis Centers: A Systematic Review and Meta-Analysis." *JAMA* 288, no. 19 (November 2002): 2449–57.

Devers, Kelly, and Robert Berenson. "Can Accountable Care Organizations Improve the Value of Health Care by Solving the Cost and Quality Quandaries?" *Timely Analysis of Immediate Health Policy Issues*, October 2009.

Dodd, J. M., C. A. Crowther, R. M. Grivell, and A. R. Deussen. "Elective Repeat Caesarean Section versus Induction of Labour for Women with a Previous Caesarean Birth." *Cochrane Database of Systematic Reviews* 12 (2014): CD004906.

Down, Simon. *Narratives of Enterprise: Crafting Entrepreneurial Self-Identity in a Small Firm.* Northampton, MA: Edward Elgar, 2006.

Feemster, Laura C., and David H. Au. "Penalizing Hospitals for Chronic Obstructive Pulmonary Disease Readmissions." *American Journal of Respiratory and Critical Care Medicine* 189, no. 6 (2014): 634–39.

Feldman, Martha S. *Order without Design: Information Production and Policy Making.* Stanford, CA: Stanford University Press, 1989.

Fine, Gary Alan, and David Shulman. "Lies from the Field: Ethical Issues in Organizational Ethnography." In *Organizational Ethnography: Studying the Complexities of Everyday Life,* edited by Sierk Ybema, Dvora Yanow, Harry Wels, and Frans Kamsteeg, 177–95. Los Angeles: Sage, 2009.

Fisher, Elliott S., Stephen M. Shortell, Sara A. Kreindler, Aricca D. Van Citters, and Bridget K. Larson. "A Framework for Evaluating the Formation, Implementation, and Performance of Accountable Care Organizations." *Health Affairs* 31, no. 11 (November 2012): 2368–78.

Flavin, Jeanne. *Our Bodies, Our Crimes: The Policing of Women's Reproduction in America.* New York: New York University Press, 2009.

"Fleecing Hospitals to Fix State Budget." *The Day,* March 10, 2013.

Folkemer, Donna C., Laura A. Spicer, Carl H. Mueller, Martha H. Somerville, Avery L. R. Brow Jr., Charles J. Milligan, and Cynthia L. Boddie-Willis. "Hospital Community Benefits after the ACA: The Emerging Federal Framework." *Issue Brief,* January 2011.

Foner, Nancy. *The Caregiving Dilemma: Work in an American Nursing Home.* Berkeley: University of California Press, 1994.

Galewitz, Phil. "Not a Hospital, Not a Home Birth: The Rise of the Birth Center." *CNN,* October 12, 2015.

Gimovsky, A. C., and V. Berghella. "Randomized Controlled Trial of Prolonged Second Stage: Extending the Time Limit vs. Usual Guidelines." *American Journal of Obstetrics and Gynecology* 214, no. 3 (March 2016): 361.e1–6.

Gold, Jenny. "Accountable Care Organizations, Explained." *NPR,* January 18, 2011.

———. "Mergers of For-Profit, Non-Profit Hospitals: How Does It Help?" *USA Today,* July 13, 2010.

Goldsmith, Jeff. "Accountable Care Organizations: The Case for Flexible Partnerships between Health Plans and Providers." *Health Affairs* 30, no. 1 (January 2011): 32–40.

Goldsmith, Jeff, and Nathan Koffman. "Pioneer ACOs: Anatomy of a 'Victory.'" *Health Affairs Blog* (blog), June 18, 2015. http://healthaffairs.org/blog/.

Goodman, John. "Six Problems with the ACA That Aren't Going Away." *Health Affairs Blog* (blog), June 25, 2015. http://healthaffairs.org/blog/.

Gouldner, Alvin Ward. *Patterns of Industrial Bureaucracy.* New York: Free Press, 1965.

Grootscholten, K., M. Kok, S. G. Oei, B. W. Mol, and J. A. van der Post. "External Cephalic Version-Related Risks: A Meta-Analysis." *Obstetrics and Gynecology* 112, no. 5 (November 2008): 1143–51.

Haar, Dan. "Hope for a Revival of Axiom Hospital Deal." *Hartford Courant,* January 5, 2015.

———. "Malloy to Axiom: Let's Make This Hospital Merger Work." *Hartford Courant,* January 12, 2015.

Hamilton, Brady E., Joyce A. Martin, Michelle J. K. Osterman Anne K. Driscoll, and Lauren M. Rossen. "Births: Provisional Data for 2016." *Vital Statistics Rapid Release* 2 (June 2017): 1–21.

Harper, L. M., A. G. Cahill, S. Boslaugh, A. O. Odibo, D. M. Stamilio, K. A. Roehl, and G. A. Macones. "Association of Induction of Labor and Uterine Rupture in Women Attempting Vaginal Birth after Cesarean: A Survival Analysis." *American Journal of Obstetrics and Gynecology* 206, no. 1 (January 2012): 51.e1–5.

Hartocollis, Anemona. "2 Hospital Networks Agree to Merge, Raising Specter of Costlier Care." *New York Times,* July 16, 2013.

Hochschild, Arlie Russell. *The Managed Heart: Commercialization of Human Feeling.* 20th anniv. ed. Berkeley: University of California Press, 2003.

Hodnett, E. D., S. Gates, G. J. Hofmeyr, and C. Sakala. "Continuous Support for Women during Childbirth." *Cochrane Database of Systematic Reviews* 7 (2015): CD003766.

Horwitz, Jill. "The ACA's Hospital Tax-Exemption Rules and the Practice of Medicine." *Health Affairs Blog* (blog), March 3, 2015. http://healthaffairs.org/blog/.

———. "Does Nonprofit Ownership Matter?" *Yale Journal on Regulation* 24, no. 1 (2007): 139–204.

Howley, Patrick. "Obamacare Installs New Scrutiny, Fines for Charitable Hospitals That Treat Uninsured People." *Daily Caller,* August 8, 2013.

Jacovino, Ed. "Axiom's Way Eased." *Journal Inquirer,* May 8, 2014.

——— "Bill Vetoed That Would Have Allowed More for Profits to Buy Hospitals." *Journal Inquirer,* July 12, 2013.

———. "DHN Picks Suitor." *Journal Inquirer,* August 9, 2013.

———. "Malloy Signs Bill Aiding DHN Sale." *Journal Inquirer,* June 4, 2014.

Jaffee, David. *Organization Theory: Tension and Change.* Boston: McGraw-Hill, 2001.

Johnson, Kelley. *Deinstitutionalising Women: An Ethnographic Study of Institutional Closure.* New York: Cambridge University Press, 1998.

Joynt, Karen E., and Ashish K. Jha. "Thirty-Day Readmissions: Truth and Consequences." *New England Journal of Medicine* 366, no. 15 (2012): 1366–69.

Jozwiak, Marta, and Jodie M. Dodd. "Methods of Term Labour Induction for Women with a Previous Caesarean Section." *Cochrane Database of Systematic Reviews* 3 (2013): 1–22.

Kahn, Charles N., Thomas Ault, Lisa Potetz, Thomas Walke, Jayne Hart Chambers, and Samantha Burch. "Assessing Medicare's Hospital Pay-for-Performance Programs and Whether They Are Achieving Their Goals." *Health Affairs* 34, no. 8 (August 2015): 1281–88.

Kavanagh, Kevin T., Jeannie P. Cimiotti, Said Abusalem, and Mary-Beth Coty. "Moving Healthcare Quality Forward with Nursing-Sensitive Value-Based Purchasing." *Journal of Nursing Scholarship* 44, no. 4 (2012): 385–95.

Keating, Christopher. "Hospitals Go Head-to-Head with Malloy; Running Biggest Media Campaign in More Than 30 Years." *Hartford Courant,* December 1, 2015.

Kintz, Diane Lindo. "Nursing Support in Labor." *Journal of Obstetric, Gynecologic, and Neonatal Nursing* 16, no. 2 (1987): 126–30.

Klein, Robert P., Nancy Fohrell Gist, Joanne Nicholson, and Kay Standley. "A Study of Father and Nurse Support during Labor." *Birth* 8, no. 3 (1981): 161–64.

Kocher, Robert, and Nikhil R. Sahni. "Hospitals' Race to Employ Physicians: The Logic behind a Money-Losing Proposition." *New England Journal of Medicine* 364, no. 19 (2011): 1790–93.

Kozhimannil, K. B., M. R. Law, and B. A. Virnig. "Cesarean Delivery Rates Vary Tenfold among U.S. Hospitals; Reducing Variation May Address Quality and Cost Issues." *Health Affairs (Millwood)* 32, no. 3 (March 2013): 527–35.

Kunda, Gideon. *Engineering Culture: Control and Commitment in a High-Tech Corporation.* Rev. ed. Philadelphia: Temple University Press, 2006.

Kurtz, Steven M., Edmund C. Lau, Kevin L. Ong, Edward M. Adler, Frank R. Kolisek, and Michael T. Manley. "Hospital, Patient, and Clinical Factors Influence 30- and 90-Day Readmission after Primary Total Hip Arthroplasty." *Journal of Arthroplasty* 31, no. 10 (2016): 2130–38.

———. "Which Clinical and Patient Factors Influence the National Economic Burden of Hospital Readmissions after Total Joint Arthroplasty?" *Clinical Orthopaedics and Related Research*, January 20, 2017.

Kurtzman, Ellen T., Ellen M. Dawson, and Jean E. Johnson. "The Current State of Nursing Performance Measurement, Public Reporting, and Value-Based Purchasing." *Policy, Politics, and Nursing Practice* 9, no. 3 (August 2008): 181–91.

Latour, Bruno, and Steve Woolgar. *Laboratory Life: The Social Construction of Scientific Facts.* Beverly Hills, CA: Sage, 1979.

Law, John. *Organizing Modernity.* Oxford, UK: Blackwell, 1994.

Leveno, K. J., D. B. Nelson, and D. D. McIntire. "Second-Stage Labor: How Long Is Too Long?" *American Journal of Obstetrics and Gynecology* 214, no. 4 (April 2016): 484–89.

Livingston, Gretchen, and D'Vera Cohn. "Childless up among All Women; Down among Women with Advanced Degrees." In *Social and Demographic Trends,* 1–8. Washington, DC: Pew Research Center, 2010.

Lundberg, George A. F. *Fuller Hospital: The First 75 Years.* Manchester, CT: Grames Printing, 2012.

MacDorman, Marian, and Eugene Declercq. "Trends in United States Out-of-Hospital Births, 2004–2014: New Information on Risk Status and Access to Care." *Birth* 43, no. 2 (June 2016): 16–124.

Madoff, Ray D. "How the Government Gives." *New York Times,* December 6, 2013.

Main, Elliott, Christine H. Morton, David Hopkins, Giovanna Giuliani, Kathryn Melsop, and Jeffrey Gould. "Cesarean Deliveries, Outcomes, and Opportunities for Change in California: Toward a Public Agenda for Maternity Care Safety and Quality." In *CMQCC White Paper,* edited by California Maternal Quality Care Collaborative, 1–86. Stanford, CA: CMQCC, 2011.

Martin, Karin A. "Giving Birth Like a Girl." *Gender and Society* 17, no. 1 (2003): 54–72.

McWilliams, J. Michael, Michael E. Chernew, Bruce E. Landon, and Aaron L. Schwartz. "Performance Differences in Year 1 of Pioneer Accountable Care Organizations." *New England Journal of Medicine* 372, no. 20 (2015): 1927–36.

McWilliams, J. Michael, and Zirui Song. "Implications for ACOs of Variations in Spending Growth." *New England Journal of Medicine* 366, no. 19 (2012): e29.

Mello, M. M., A. Kachalia, and D. M. Studdert. "Administrative Compensation for Medical Injuries: Lessons from Three Foreign Systems." *Issue Brief (Commonw Fund)* 14 (July 2011): 1–18.

Mello, M. M., D. M. Studdert, and A. Kachalia. "The Medical Liability Climate and Prospects for Reform." *JAMA* 312, no. 20 (November 2014): 2146–55.

Mello, Michelle M., David M. Studdert, Allen B. Kachalia, and Troyen A. Brennan. "'Health Courts' and Accountability for Patient Safety." *Milbank Quarterly* 84, no. 3 (2006): 459–92.

Michak, Don. "Axiom Calls It Quits." *Journal Inquirer*, February 5, 2015.

———. "Axiom Denies Layoff Role." *Journal Inquirer*, October 24, 2014.

———. "Axiom Gives Malloy Terms to Revive Hospital Buyout Plans." *Journal Inquirer*, January 22, 2015.

———. "Axiom's Way around Governor's Veto Is Elite University." *Journal Inquirer*, November 19, 2013.

———. "Deadline Extended for DHN and Waranoke." *Journal Inquirer*, October 14, 2015.

———. "DHN Blames State Cuts for Wage Freeze, Stops Retirement Account Contributions." *Journal Inquirer*, November 5, 2015.

———. "DHN Faces 'Extraordinary Challenges.'" *Journal Inquirer*, October 23, 2014.

———. "DHN Hospitalist Company Used by Axiom." *Journal Inquirer*, March 24, 2014.

———. "DHN Hospitals Lag on Financial Measures for Third Consecutive Year." *Journal Inquirer*, August 25, 2015.

———. "DHN Sheds More Jobs." *Journal Inquirer*, July 15, 2015.

———. "DHN's New Suitor Owned by a Buyout Firm." *Journal Inquirer*, June 26, 2015.

———. "The Doctor Is Out—West." *Journal Inquirer*, October 23, 2013.

———. "Execs Loot DHN on Eve of Sale." *Journal Inquirer*, October 24, 2015.

———. "Unionized DHN Employees Trade Contract Concessions for Job Security." *Journal Inquirer*, November 25, 2014.

Michak, Don, and John Kennedy. "Approved but Not OK; DHN Hospital Sales Questioned." *Journal Inquirer*, April 30, 2014.

Michak, Don, and Mike Savino. "DHN Pleads for Help." *Journal Inquirer*, December 23, 2014.

Miller, Jake. "Inside Health-Reform Savings: Details of Early Savings by Medicare Pioneer ACO Program Point Ways to Improvement." *Harvard Medical School*, April 15, 2015. http://hms.harvard.edu/.

Moeran, Brian. *Ethnography at Work*. New York: Berg, 2006.

Morris, Theresa. *Cut It Out: The C-Section Epidemic in America*. Rev. ed. New York: NYU Press, 2016.

Morris, Theresa, and Katherine McInerney. "Media Representations of Pregnancy and Childbirth: An Analysis of Reality Television Programs in the United States." *Birth* 37, no. 2 (June 2010): 134–40.

Morris, Theresa, Kelly McNamara, and Christine H. Morton. "Hospital-Ownership and Cesareans in the United States." Birth (forthcoming).

Morris, Theresa, Olivia Meredith, Mia Schulman, and Christine Morton. "Why Do Low-Risk Women Have C-Sections? A Case Study of a Tertiary Care Hospital." *Women's Health Issues* 26, no. 3 (2015): 329–35.

Morris, Theresa, and Joan H. Robinson. "Forced and Coerced Cesarean Sections in the United States." Contexts 16, no. 2 (Spring 2017): 24–29.

Morris, Theresa, and Mia Schulman. "Race Inequality in Epidural Use and Regional Anesthesia Failure in Labor and Birth: An Examination of Women's Experience." *Sexual and Reproductive Healthcare* 5, no. 4 (December 2014): 188–94.

Mrozinski, Josh. "Purchase of Mercy Hospital Could Return Nearly $1 Million to Local Tax Rolls." *Scranton Times-Tribune*, February 12, 2011.

Muhlestein, David. "Growth and Dispersion of Accountable Care Organizations in 2015." *Health Affairs Blog* (blog), March 31, 2015. http://healthaffairs.org/blog/.

Muhlestein, David, and Mark McClellan. "Accountable Care Organizations in 2016: Private and Public-Sector Growth and Dispersion." *Health Affairs Blog* (blog), April 21, 2016. http://healthaffairs.org/blog/.

O'Brien, Joseph A., Jr. "Marple Hospital to Eliminate Childbirth Services." *Hartford Courant*, November 2, 2010.

O'Connor, N. R., K. O. Tanabe, M. S. Siadaty, and F. R. Hauck. "Pacifiers and Breast-feeding: A Systematic Review." *Archives of Pediatrics and Adolescent Medicine* 163, no. 4 (April 2009): 378–82.

Ogasawara, Yuko. *Office Ladies and Salaried Men: Power, Gender, and Work in Japanese Companies*. Berkeley: University of California Press, 1998.

Ohlsson, Arne, and Vibhuti S. Shah. "Intrapartum Antibiotics for Known Maternal Group B Streptococcal Colonization." *Cochrane Database of Systematic Reviews* 6 (2014): 1–45.

Pazniokas, Mark. "Axiom Ends Bid to Acquire Connecticut Hospitals." *Hartford Courant*, December 11, 2014.

———. "Battle Lines Drawn over Conditions on Waterbury Hospital Deal." *Hartford Courant*, December 10, 2014.

Perrow, Charles. "A Society of Organizations." *Theory and Society* 20, no. 6 (1991): 725–62.

Pfeffer, Jeffrey. *Power in Organizations*. Marshfield, MA: Pitman, 1981.

———. "You're Still the Same: Why Theories of Power Hold over Time and across Contexts." *Academy of Management Perspectives* 27, no. 4 (November 2013): 269–80.

Pfeffer, Jeffrey, and Gerald R Salancik. *The External Control of Organizations: A Resource Dependence Perspective*. Stanford, CA: Stanford University Press, 2003.

Phaneuf, Keith M. "Defying Malloy, Legislators Pitch a $1.8 Billion Revenue Increase." *Connecticut Mirror*, April 29, 2015.

Phaneuf, Keith M., and Mark Pazniokas. "Lembo Joins Dissent over Malloy's Emergency Budget Cuts." *Connecticut Mirror*, October 1, 2015.

Phipps-Taylor, Madeleine, and the West Coast Harkness Policy Forum. "Getting to the ACO Tipping Point: What Else Might Be Needed?" *Health Affairs Blog* (blog), June 3, 2015. http://healthaffairs.org/blog/.

Prechel, Harland. "Historical Contingency Theory, Policy Paradigm Shifts, and Corporate Malfeasance at the Turn of the 21st Century." *Political Sociology for the 21st Century* 12 (2003): 311–40.

———. "Irrationality and Contradiction in Organizational Change: Transformation in the Corporate Form of a U.S. Steel Corporation, 1930–1987." *Sociological Quarterly* 32, no. 3 (1991): 423–45.

Prechel, Harland, and Theresa Morris. "The Effects of Organizational and Political Embeddedness on Financial Malfeasance in the Largest U.S. Corporations: Dependence, Incentives, and Opportunities." *American Sociological Review* 75, no. 3 (June 2010): 331–54.

Prechel, Harland, Theresa Morris, Tim Woods, and Rachel Walden. "Corporate Diversification Revisited: The Political-Legal Environment, the Multilayer-Subsidiary Form, and Mergers and Acquisitions." *Sociological Quarterly* 49, no. 4 (2008): 849–78.

Prince, Cathryn J. "Battle Emerging over Proposed Tax on Nonprofit Hospitals." *Connecticut Patch*, March 28, 2011.

Radin, T. G., J. S. Harmon, and D. A. Hanson. "Nurses' Care during Labor: Its Effect on the Cesarean Birth Rate of Healthy, Nulliparous Women." *Birth* 20, no. 1 (March 1993): 14–21.

Radnofsky, Louise. "How the ACA May Affect Health Costs: Some Provisions Have Taken Effect, but Others Won't Kick in for Several Years." *Wall Street Journal*, February 23, 2014.

Ragin, Charles C. *The Comparative Method: Moving beyond Qualitative and Quantitative Strategies*. Berkeley: University of California Press, 1987.

Richman, B. D., and K. A. Schulman. "A Cautious Path Forward on Accountable Care Organizations." *JAMA* 305, no. 6 (2011): 602–3.

Roberts, J. E. "Factors Influencing Distress from Pain during Labor." *MCN: The American Journal of Maternal/Child Nursing* 8, no. 1 (January/February 1983): 62–66.

Rosenbaum, Sara. "Additional Requirements for Charitable Hospitals: Final Rules on Community Health Needs Assessments and Financial Assistance." *Health Affairs Blog* (blog), January 23, 2015. http://healthaffairs.org/blog/.

———. "Tax-Exempt Status for Nonprofit Hospitals under the ACA: Where Are the Final Treasury/IRS Rules?" *Health Affairs Blog* (blog), October 23, 2014. http://healthaffairs.org/blog/.

Rosenberg, Tina. "Reducing Unnecessary C-Section Births." *New York Times Opinionator* (blog), January 16, 2016. http://opinionator.blogs.nytimes.com/.

Rostow, Victoria P., and Roger J. Bulger, eds. *Medical Professional Liability and the Delivery of Obstetrical Care: Volume II, an Interdisciplinary Review*. Washington, DC: National Academies Press, 1989.

Rudowitz, Robin. "Issue Brief: How Do Medicaid Disproportionate Share Hospital (DSH) Payments Change under the ACA?" *Henry J. Kaiser Family Foundation*, November 18, 2013.

Salancik, Gerald R., and Jeffrey Pfeffer. "Who Gets Power—and How They Hold on to It: A Strategic-Contingency Model of Power." *Organizational Dynamics* 5, no. 3 (1977): 3–21.

Segal, Mike. "Quality/Cost Initiative of PPACA: An Evolution in Healthcare Delivery?" *Journal of Medical Practice Management* 26, no. 2 (2010): 106–8.

Selznick, Philip. *TVA and the Grass Roots: A Study in the Sociology of Formal Organization.* Berkeley: University of California Press, 1949.

Shields, Donna. "Nursing Care in Labour and Patient Satisfaction: A Descriptive Study." *Journal of Advanced Nursing* 3, no. 6 (November 1978): 535–50.

Shortell, Stephen M., Lawrence P. Casalino, and Elliott S. Fisher. "How the Center for Medicare and Medicaid Innovation Should Test Accountable Care Organizations." *Health Affairs* 29, no. 7 (July 2010): 1293–98.

Smith, Pam. *The Emotional Labour of Nursing Revisited: Can Nurses Still Care?* 2nd ed. New York: Palgrave Macmillan, 2012.

Smith, Vicki. *Managing in the Corporate Interest: Control and Resistance in an American Bank.* Berkeley: University of California Press, 1990.

Sng, Ban Leong, Wan Ling Leong, Yanzhi Zeng, Fahad Javaid Siddiqui, Pryseley N. Assam, Yvonne Lim, Edwin S. Y. Chan, and Alex T. Sia. "Early versus Late Initiation of Epidural Analgesia for Labour." *Cochrane Database of Systematic Reviews* 10 (2014): 1–77.

Snowden, Jonathan M., Ellen L. Tilden, Janice Snyder, Brian Quigley, Aaron B. Caughey, and Yvonne W. Cheng. "Planned Out-of-Hospital Birth and Birth Outcomes." *New England Journal of Medicine* 373, no. 27 (2015): 2642–53.

Sommer, Jeff. "Gripes about Obamacare Aside, Health Insurers Are in a Profit Spiral." *New York Times*, March 18, 2017.

Soper, Kim. "Directional Hospital System Laying Off Managers while Negotiating Nurses Contract." *Journal Inquirer*, October 18, 2014.

———. "Safety Grade Slips for Hospitals." *Journal Inquirer*, April 30, 2016.

Spong, C. Y., V. Berghella, K. D. Wenstrom, B. M. Mercer, and G. R. Saade. "Preventing the First Cesarean Delivery: Summary of a Joint Eunice Kennedy Shriver National Institute of Child Health and Human Development, Society for Maternal-Fetal Medicine, and American College of Obstetricians and Gynecologists Workshop." *Obstetrics and Gynecology* 120, no. 5 (November 2012): 1181–93.

Stankiewicz, Jonathan M. "Directional Health System Corporators OK Sale." *Journal Inquirer*, May 13, 2014.

Stapleton, S. R., C. Osborne, and J. Illuzzi. "Outcomes of Care in Birth Centers: Demonstration of a Durable Model." *Journal of Midwifery and Women's Health* 58, no. 1 (January/February 2013): 3–14.

Starr, Paul. *Remedy and Reaction: The Peculiar American Struggle over Healthcare Reform.* Rev. ed. New Haven, CT: Yale University Press, 2013.

———. *The Social Transformation of American Medicine.* New York: Basic Books, 1982.

Stefan, M. S., P. S. Pekow, W. Nsa, A. Priya, L. E. Miller, D. W. Bratzler, M. B. Rothberg, et al. "Hospital Performance Measures and 30-Day Readmission Rates." *Journal of General Internal Medicine* 28, no. 3 (March 2013): 377–85.

Stevens, Bonnie, Janet Yamada, Grace Y. Lee, and Arne Ohlsson. "Sucrose for Analgesia in Newborn Infants Undergoing Painful Procedures." *Cochrane Database of Systematic Reviews* 1 (2013): 1–355.

Sturdevant, Matthew. "Axiom CEO Skewers Regulatory Environment, but Is Open to a Deal." *Hartford Courant*, January 22, 2015.

———. "Axiom Declines to Comment on Malloy Letter." *Hartford Courant*, January 13, 2015.

———. "State Regulators Approve Joint Venture of Axiom, Waterbury Hospital, with Conditions." *Hartford Courant*, December 1, 2014.

Sturdevant, Matthew, and Christopher Keating. "Axiom's Plan to Buy Connecticut Hospitals Is Dead." *Hartford Courant*, February 5, 2015.

Sweha, A., T. W. Hacker, and J. Nuovo. "Interpretation of the Electronic Fetal Heart Rate during Labor." *American Family Physician* 59, no. 9 (May 1999): 2487–500.

Taubenberger, Jeffery K., and David M. Morens. "1918 Influenza: The Mother of All Pandemics." *Emerging Infectious Diseases* 12, no. 1 (2006): 15–22.

Tavernise, Sabrian. "Maternal Mortality Rate in U.S. Rises, Defying Global Trend, Study Finds." *New York Times*, September 21, 2016.

Uberoi, Namrata, Kenneth Finegold, and Emily Gee. "Health Insurance Coverage and the Affordable Care Act, 2010–2016." *ASPE Issue Brief*, March 2016.

U.S. Department of Health and Human Services. "2011 Report to Congress: National Strategy for Quality Improvement in Health Care." In *Working for Quality*. Washington, DC: Agency for Healthcare Research and Quality, 2011.

Vigdor, Neil. "Malloy Stays the Course with Controversial Plan to Tax Hospitals." *Stamford Advocate*, February 13, 2011.

Vogt, William B., and Robert Town. "How Has Hospital Consolidation Affected the Price and Quality of Hospital Care?" *Synthesis Project*, February 2006.

Watson, Tony J. *In Search of Management: Culture, Chaos and Control in Managerial Work*. Rev. ed. London: Thomas Learning, 2001.

Weick, Karl E. *The Social Psychology of Organizing*. 2nd ed. Reading, MA: Addison-Wesley, 1979.

Weisman, Robert. "Equity Firm Set to Buy Caritas." *Boston Globe*, March 25, 2010.

Werner, Rachel M., and R. Adams Dudley. "Medicare's New Hospital Value-Based Purchasing Program Is Likely to Have Only a Small Impact on Hospital Payments." *Health Affairs* 31, no. 9 (September 2012): 1932–40.

Wolcott, Harry F. *The Man in the Principal's Office: An Ethnography*. Rev. ed. Walnut Creek, CA: AltaMira Press, 2003.

Wolosin, Robert, Louis Ayala, and Bradley R. Fulton. "Nursing Care, Inpatient Satisfaction, and Value-Based Purchasing: Vital Connections." *Journal of Nursing Administration* 42, no. 6 (2012): 321–25.

Zabusky, Stacia E. *Launching Europe: An Ethnography of European Cooperation in Space Science*. Princeton, NJ: Princeton University Press, 1995.

Zald, Mayer N. *Organizational Change: The Political Economy of the YMCA*. Chicago: University of Chicago Press, 1970.

INDEX

abortion access, 202

Abrams, Melinda, 172, 182

ACA (Affordable Care Act; Obamacare), 172–83; Accountable Care Organizations, 177–79, 182–83, 201; bundled payments under, 176–77; critiques of, 18, 172; distrust of hospitals and health-care providers in, 202; effect on hospitals, 182–83, 189–91, 196–97; effect on patient care, 198; goals of, 2–3, 172; health insurance companies' profits under, 172; hospitals pressured by, 131, 184–85, 196; Medicare funding under, 141, 196; Medicare/Medicaid reimbursements under, 172, 180–81; Medicare readmission rates under, 173–74, 191–92, 196; merger incentive under, 181–82; non-profit hospital status under, 179–82; obstetrical (OB) nurses affected by, 1–2; pay-for-performance programs in, 173–76; and state-level policies, 171, 183–93

Accountable Care Organizations (ACOs), 177–79, 182–83, 201

Affordable Care Act. See ACA

Anderson, Claudia, 6

anesthesiologists, 141, 197, 210n1

Arnold, Jill, 200–201

Association of periOperative Registered Nurses (AORN), 45

Association of Women's Health, Obstetric and Neonatal Nurses (AWHONN), 90

Berenson, Robert, 183

birth ball, 54, 86, 88

birth centers, 200, 221n10

birthing rooms, 195

BirthNetwork National, 199

Blumenthal, David, 172, 182

breastfeeding: colostrum during, 122; LATCH assessment of, 59; nurses' help with, 59, 122, 145, 156–57, 159, 211n7; and pacifiers, 123

Bundled Payments for Care Improvement, 176–77

case-study methodology, 10–16

catheterization, intermittent ("straight cath"), 95, 105–6, 213n13

cephalopelvic disproportion (CPD), 81

cesareans: for breech presentation, 104; data on, 200–201; forced, 202; labor before, 134; for multiple births, 133; rates of, 7, 10–11, 209n44. See also VBACs

charge nurses, 36–38, 41, 43–44, 90, 133, 162

CHNA requirements, 179–80

circulator nurses, 35, 210n1

circumcision, 48–49, 59, 95–96

Congressional Budget Office, 2–3

Consumer Reports, 200–201

CPMs (certified professional midwives), 200, 221n11

custodians, 73–76, 159, 161–62

Cut It Out: The C-Section Epidemic in United States (Morris), 3–4

Cytotec, 98

ABOUT THE AUTHOR

Theresa Morris is Associate Professor of Sociology at Texas A&M University, where she teaches courses on organizations, gender, reproduction, and research methods. She is the author of *Cut It Out: The Cesarean Epidemic in America* (NYU Press, 2013).